ANTABUSE TREATMENT FOR ALCOHOLISM:
AN EVIDENCE-BASED HANDBOOK FOR MEDICAL
AND NON-MEDICAL CLINICIANS.

ANTABUSE TREATMENT FOR ALCOHOLISM: AN EVIDENCE-BASED HANDBOOK FOR MEDICAL AND NON-MEDICAL CLINICIANS.

Why supervised disulfiram is more effective than other drugs for alcoholism and how to integrate it with psycho-social interventions to achieve lasting abstinence or controlled drinking.

By
Colin Brewer and Emmanuel Streel

Note: We have tried to ensure that all information in this book is accurate at the time of publication but we neither provide nor imply any guarantees as to its completeness or reliability. Websites listed in this book may change. This book is not intended to be a substitute for medical advice from a licensed physician. Readers should consult their doctors about any matters relating to their own health.

Copyright © 2018 – Colin Brewer

Contents

- FOREWORD by William R Miller.

- PREFACE

- Chapter 1 The Origins Of Disulfiram Treatment: A Tale Of Serendipity, Rubber And War, In Which No Animals Were Harmed. 1-8

- Chapter 2 The Importance Of Supervised Consumption, Family Involvement, Problem-Oriented Therapies And Formal Or Informal Treatment Contracts. 9-18

- Chapter 3 The Misleading 'Randomized Controlled Trials' Of Disulfiram. 19-24

- Chapter 4 The Japanese Connection. 27-32

- Chapter 5 The Varieties Of Alcoholic Experience. 33-42

- Chapter 6 Disulfiram's Role In Retaining Ambivalent Patients In Treatment And Identifying The Unmotivated. 43-48

- Chapter 7 Components Of Effectiveness In Disulfiram Treatment And Other Interventions For Alcoholism – Including Placebo And Non-Specific Effects. 49-62

- Chapter 8 International Experts Who Routinely Use Disulfiram. Proceedings of the Copenhagen round-table Disulfiram symposium of 1996. 63-106

- Chapter 9 Initiating Disulfiram Treatment: Some Basic Practices And Principles. 107-118

- Chapter 10 Supervision in The Context Of Probation And Parole. Dealing with recurrent alcoholic offenders. 119-132

- Chapter 11 How Disulfiram Facilitates Psychosocial Interventions And Rehabilitation: the language-learning analogy, the OLITA programme, and its 9-year follow-up. 133-147

- Chapter 12 A Counter-Intuitive Application: Using Disulfiram In Controlled Drinking Programmes. 149-158

- Chapter 13 Disulfiram Treatment In Special Populations. 159-169

- Chapter 14 'Safer Than Aspirin': The Side-Effects Of Disulfiram. 171-192

- Chapter 15 The Ethics, Philosophy And Politics Of Disulfiram Treatment. 193-206

- Chapter 16 The Implications Of Disulfiram's Effectiveness And Modes Of Action For The

Hypothesis That 'Addiction Is A Chronic Brain Disease'. 207-214

- Chapter 17 Disulfiram vs. Other Medications for Alcoholism. 215-226

- Chapter 18 Why Can't We Have a Disulfiram Implant? 227-233

- Chapter 19:Disulfiram, The Japanese (Again) and The Potential Of Gene Therapy. 235-238

- Chapter 20 Conclusion. 239-242

- Appendix 1. Other Uses Of Disulfiram.

- Appendix 2. (Viewable on the website at planetservetus.org) Fear And Loathing In Westminster

- Acknowledgements

FOREWORD

William R. Miller, Ph.D.
Emeritus Distinguished Professor of Psychology and Psychiatry
The University of New Mexico, USA

What has kept me engaged in this field for more than forty years now is that the outcomes of treatment for alcohol use disorders are so good. Over the years our team has had had the privilege of following everyone participating in our clinical trials, and contrary to public opinion, most people treated for alcohol problems do get well. We are blessed, really, with a large and growing family of scientifically proven tools to help people escape the slippery slope of problematic drinking and dependence.

Disulfiram has been something of a stepchild in this family of effective options. Now a mature adult, this stepchild has long been there in the background but often ignored and underappreciated. Some don't even know its name, but it has endured the relegation and remains a valuable member of the family.

Beyond the outcome research reviewed in this book, disulfiram has much to recommend it. Primary care providers can prescribe it, and it is easy to use. It is a relatively simple, inexpensive, and well-understood medication. Taken faithfully in adequate dosage, it effectively suppresses alcohol use and gives the person a head start on sobriety. It is easily combined with other forms of treatment such as the community reinforcement approach. As with many medications, the primary obstacle to effectiveness has been adherence, an issue well recognized and addressed in this volume by Brewer and Streel. Particularly with available supports for adherence, disulfiram is a valuable and effective treatment tool.

It is puzzling why this useful tool has been so underutilized. Fortunes have been poured into developing, testing, marketing, and buying alternative medications with modest efficacy. There has been substantial progress in screening and brief treatment for alcohol problems in primary health care, but utilization of disulfiram remains low. I am pleased, therefore, to see this important textbook encouraging and informing the use of disulfiram in treating alcohol problems – the first such professional volume in thirty years. No single method is appropriate for everyone with alcohol use disorders but disulfiram deserves a place in the family.

PREFACE

One reason for writing this book is a story told to us in 2016 by a London NHS GP who had started a successfully detoxified alcoholic patient on disulfiram – better known by its trade-name *Antabuse* - before referring him to an alcoholism service linked to the world-famous local teaching hospital for the intensive psychological support and treatment that he clearly needed as well. A day after the patient's first appointment, the nurse who had interviewed him there telephoned the GP. "I'm very interested in this drug you prescribed for him," she said "but I've not come across it before. It sounds a good idea and I'd like to discuss it with the rest of the team. Can you tell me a bit about it?" This book is intended in part for the apparently large number of non-physician alcoholism clinicians – nurses, clinical psychologists and counsellors - who, like that nurse, don't know much about disulfiram but think it sounds a good idea and would like to know more. It is also intended for physicians who are interested in treating their alcoholic patients, whether as gastroenterologists, cardiologists, general psychiatrists or GPs – especially GPs. And, of course, alcoholism or general addiction specialists. For all these doctors, the ravages of alcoholism are a regular challenge and an important cause of premature death but many of them do not realise how disulfiram can make it much easier for them (and their patients) to meet that challenge.

Another reason is that while there are many textbooks on alcoholism treatment, few of them give the space and prominence to disulfiram that its effectiveness merits. Only a single textbook devoted to disulfiram seems to have been written.[1] It was published in 1987 and while it contains much clinical experience and many useful and recondite references to older publications, it is now both out of date and out of print.[2] Until well into the 1990s, textbooks that did mention disulfiram often failed to mention the crucial importance of supervised consumption and many literature reviews – more up-to-date than textbooks – even questioned its effectiveness. Only in the last decade has that disparagement begun to change.

To paraphrase the great 17th century English physician and sceptic Thomas Sydenham: "Among the remedies which it has pleased Almighty God to give to man to relieve his sufferings, few have been so underused and so misunderstood as disulfiram".[3] In this book, we aim to explain how disulfiram works – and almost equally importantly, how it does *not* work - and to set out the evidence from individual studies and from meta-analyses that show disulfiram to be more than just slightly superior to the other drugs (acamprosate and naltrexone or nalmefene) currently licensed in most developed countries for alcoholism. With the aid of case-histories, we show how its uptake and effectiveness can be maximised and most usefully

---

[1] McNichol R, Ewing J, Faiman M. Disulfiram (Antabuse) A unique medical aid to sobriety. Springfield. Charles Thomas. 1987

[2] For some reason, many pages are printed entirely in block capitals, which makes them difficult to read.

[3] Sydenham's original epigram was: 'Among the remedies which it has pleased Almighty God to give to man to relieve his sufferings, none is so efficacious as opium'. Opium, even in its natural form, is still an effective and indispensable medicine.

combined with the problem-oriented psychosocial interventions that many – but not all – patients also need. While disulfiram is by far the best drug we have for helping heavy-drinking patients to abstain, rather than drink less heavily, it is a very flexible and adaptable intervention that can even help a useful proportion of patients to become controlled drinkers. It can also be adapted to suit the needs of special patient groups, such as recurrent alcoholic offenders, alcoholic methadone maintenance patients, and detoxified opiate abusers who drink heavily despite taking naltrexone to prevent relapse to opiates, as well as alcoholic physicians, pilots and other professionals in sensitive employments. Disulfiram is much safer – especially in comparison with continued heavy drinking - than many of its critics claim. Although it has little bearing on the management of individual patients, we discuss the philosophical and practical implications for alcoholism treatment and research – and addiction treatment and research in general - of disulfiram's superior effectiveness. This inevitably includes some quasi-political examinations of the reasons for its neglect. Since disulfiram is also being used or studied for its effectiveness in several conditions very far removed from alcoholism, an appendix gives a brief summary of these developments.

In Sydenham's day, it was no doubt true, as he claimed, that "the arrival of a good clown exercises more beneficial influence upon the health of a town than of twenty asses laden with drugs". Like Sydenham, we are instinctively sceptical - as medical scientists should be - about claims for therapeutic effectiveness, most of which have historically proved to be unfounded or greatly exaggerated. The null hypothesis – the major philosophical basis of the

Randomised Controlled Trial (RCT) – takes scepticism as the default position. It invites clinicians to *assume that the treatment in question is ineffective* and requires those who think we should use that treatment to provide evidence that disproves the assumption of ineffectiveness. Mere claims or assertions of effectiveness are to be ignored, however authoritative the claimant and especially if their supposed authority means no more than that they are well-known public figures. In the past hundred years, the effectiveness of drugs prescribed by doctors has greatly improved but not by as much as many of us would like to think. In alcoholism, the effectiveness of most of the recommended medications when compared with psychological treatments or placebo medication has not been impressive and there are many negative comparisons.

Disulfiram is a unique exception to this depressing list but it is also an exception in one other important respect, namely that because of its unique mode of action, it is uniquely unsuitable for comparison with placebo medication in blinded studies. We will discuss this in greater detail shortly. Here, we will just note that because disulfiram works by deterrence due to the fear of an unpleasant reaction if alcohol is consumed, placebo tablets in blinded trials have a similar deterrent effect, just as speed cameras have a deterrent effect on speeding even if they are inactive (provided, of course, that speeding drivers do not *know* that they are inactive). However, the similar effectiveness of active and inactive speed cameras does not mean that speed cameras are not worth installing or have no effect on speeding or on accident rates. Their deterrent effect is a matter of daily experience (and sometimes daily frustration) for most of us.

Apart from the previously unpublished proceedings of the 1996 Copenhagen Round Table Symposium on disulfiram, chapters are written by me with much advice and input from Emmanuel Streel, a colleague and co-author for nearly 20 years and some of the chapters include sections from what we regard as our two most important contributions to the disulfiram literature. [4,5] Both of us have considerable experience in the treatment of addictions. Before I became an addiction specialist, my background was in general psychiatry with an interest in cognitive-behavioural and family therapies and neuropsychiatry. I wrote my first paper on alcoholism in 1971 [6] and on disulfiram in 1980 but between then and 1992, I was the only British contributor to the peer-reviewed clinical disulfiram literature – a uniqueness that sometimes felt rather uncomfortable – and wrote or co-authored most of the British disulfiram papers after that year. I also helped to design the 1992 British multi-centre RCT of disulfiram.[7]

---

[4] Brewer C, Streel E. Learning the language of abstinence in addiction treatment: some similarities between relapse-prevention with disulfiram, naltrexone and other pharmacological antagonists and intensive 'immersion' methods of foreign language teaching. Substance Abuse, 2003; 24(3) 157-173.
[5] Brewer C, Streel E, Skinner M. Supervised Disulfiram's Superior Effectiveness in Alcoholism Treatment: Ethical, Methodological, and Psychological Aspects. Alcohol and Alcoholism, 2017, 1–7
[6] Brewer C. Perrett L. Brain damage due to alcohol consumption: a psychometric, air-encephalographic and EEG study. Brit J Addiction 1971;66:170-82
[7] Chick J, Gough K, Falkowski W, Kershaw P, Hore B, Mehta B, Ritson B, Ropner R, Torley D. Disulfiram treatment of alcoholism. Br J Psychiatry. 1992 Jul;161:84-9.

Emmanuel is a Belgian clinical psychologist with an interest in psychopharmacology. His background is in psychology and cognitive neuropsychology, with a PhD in biomedical sciences. An active researcher with clinical experience of adolescents and adults, he has published numerous articles and textbooks on mental health, addiction and clinical and fundamental neurosciences. We met through a shared interest in the opiate antagonist naltrexone when I was invited to lecture at the Free University of Brussels and have since collaborated on several papers and projects. In its heroin-blocking role, naltrexone has several interesting similarities to disulfiram that we also discuss. Naltrexone is available as depot and implanted formulations that are more effective than oral preparations. As yet, no similar formulation of disulfiram has shown genuine pharmacological (as opposed to placebo) effects but we describe some promising research in that area, as well as the potential of gene therapy for alcoholism that involves identical manipulations of alcohol metabolism.

STYLISTIC QUIRKS

At the risk of being thought a little old-fashioned, we generally use the words 'alcoholism' and 'alcoholic' as convenient shorthand for all forms of excessive, harmful, dependent or problematic drinking and those who regularly exhibit it. In our view, it does not matter very much to the clinician dealing with an individual patient whether the harm, the problem and the excess involve daily drinking with physical dependence, daily or frequent drinking with psychological but not physical dependence, or binge drinking at weekly or less frequent intervals. As a wise physician noted many years ago, despite many attempts to delineate differing types of alcohol abuse "the problem that all alcoholics have in common is that they drink too much"[8] and the job of clinicians is to help patients to alter their alcohol-related behavior so that they no longer drink too much, or do so very much less often.

Although women constitute more than half the world's population, most alcoholics in all societies are men – often by large margins. This is not something that men should feel proud of but partly for this reason and partly because we dislike sentences that repeatedly feature phrases like 'he or she', we use masculine pronouns and adjectives throughout. We hope that female or transgender readers will not be offended and may even take it as a compliment.

There are three broad categories of information in this book: the academic and evidence-based; case histories and the

---

[8] Lemere, F. The nature and significance of brain damage from alcoholism. Am J Psychiat 1956;113: 361–362.

fruits of clinical experience; and matters that can best be described as historical, philosophical or political. While most clinicians will be interested in the first two categories, not all of them will be interested in the third and it is therefore *printed in italics, thus*, so that readers can easily skip it if they wish. Additional information in this category and others is available on the book's website at planetservetus.org. Apart from the story of the late jazz saxophonist Stan Getz's encounters with disulfiram, I have, of course, changed the names of patients described in case histories and omitted, combined or altered clinically irrelevant but potentially identifying features.

Although psychologists, counsellors and therapists of various kinds without medical or nursing backgrounds can – and clearly do – work happily in programmes that include disulfiram without needing much general medical knowledge, I have included the occasional 'Note for the unmedical' where the information might be useful or merely interesting, such as the main serious medical complications of alcoholism. Finally, we have opted for footnotes rather than endnotes because references can more easily be identified (and followed-up where necessary) without tedious page-turning. This inevitably involves some repetition of references but it may also make them easier to remember. A full list is also available on the website and will be regularly updated.

Chapter 1. THE ORIGINS OF DISULFIRAM TREATMENT: a tale of serendipity, rubber and war, in which No Animals Were Harmed.

Disulfiram was first synthesized in 1881 by Grodzki, a Berlin chemist.[9] Twenty years later, it found a use as a vulcanising agent for hardening rubber. The first person who thought that it might be useful in alcoholism treatment was Dr E. E. Williams, a factory doctor employed by an American rubber company that used disulfiram extensively. In 1937, he published a letter in the New England Journal of Medicine[10] reporting that several employees found that if they drank alcohol, within a few minutes they developed unpleasant symptoms – mainly flushing, palpitations and nausea. A short investigation had soon confirmed that only workers in the factory who were exposed to disulfiram experienced what would eventually become known as the Disulfiram-Alcohol Reaction (DAR). That was the first episode of serendipity in the disulfiram story but Dr Williams's suggestion that it might be useful in managing alcoholism was not taken up.

The second episode occurred in Copenhagen in 1945. During the Second World War, Denmark was occupied by the Nazis and although the occupation was less vicious than in other occupied countries, the Danes experienced many hardships. One of these was an outbreak of scabies – the very itchy skin

---

[9] Grodzki M. Über äthylirte sulfoharnstoffe. Berl Deutsch Chem Ges 1881;14, 2754-2758.
[10] Williams E. Effects of alcohol on workers with carbon disulfide, J Am Med Assoc 1937;109, 1472-3

condition caused by a tiny mite, *Sarcoptes scabiei*,[11] that was easily transmitted in the relatively overcrowded and unhygienic conditions of wartime Denmark. It happens that disulfiram (and the closely related compound monosulfiram) kills the scabies mite. It is easily absorbed through the skin, hence the experience of the rubber workers, and it kills mites by binding (or *chelating*) - and thus inactivating - the small quantities of copper in the mite equivalent of haemoglobin, which transports oxygen in mites in the same way that the analogous iron-containing compound does in human red blood cells. Disulfiram was made by a Danish pharmaceutical company but just as it was thinking of marketing the drug for scabies, the war ended and with it the scabies epidemic. No drug company likes to abandon a potentially useful compound and since disulfiram was also known to kill intestinal worms by the same copper-chelating process, they decided to investigate its possible use as a vermicide (i.e. worm-killer) in both humans and farm or domestic animals. Rats and rabbits seemed to thrive when given disulfiram, so the next stage in that legally and institutionally relaxed era was for the company's chief disulfiram investigator – Erik Jacobsen - to take some himself and see if there were any side-effects. On that day, he accompanied his evening meal with his usual glass or two of Denmark's famous lager beers – whether Carlsberg or Tuborg is not recorded – and independently rediscovered disulfiram's alcohol-sensitising effect.[12]

---

[11] A fact that was discovered, thanks to the recently invented microscope, in 1687, making scabies the first human disease with a known cause.

[12] Ellis P, Dronsfield A. Antabuse's diamond anniversary: Still sparkling on? Drug Alc Rev 2013;32, 342–344

Several researchers in other countries who were studying disulfiram and analogous compounds (one of which, cyanamide, was widely used in the fertilizer industry) had also noticed their alcohol-sensitising effects and mused about their therapeutic potential in alcoholism without taking matters further. While Jacobsen also did some musing, he apparently did not think alcoholism was sufficiently common in Denmark to make it worth testing and promoting disulfiram for that purpose until, two years later, he happened to discuss his experience with a physician, Oluf Martensen-Larsen, who had some experience in treating alcoholic patients. Martensen-Larsen repeated the experiment on himself and duly experienced the DAR. In 1998, although too old to travel to the meeting, he explained in a written semi-centennial presentation to an addiction conference in the USA that to make matters trebly certain, they persuaded an unsuspecting colleague to take a dose of disulfiram and then invited him to join them for a beer-and-sandwich lunch. His reaction confirmed their suspicions and there is no record that he was lastingly annoyed by their deception. In 1948, Jacobsen and another colleague, J. Hald, published a second report of disulfiram's alcohol-sensitising effects in the Lancet[13] and in the same issue, Martensen-Larsen published the first account of the treatment of alcoholism with disulfiram.[14]

---

[13] Hald J, Jacobsen E. A drug sensitising the organism to ethyl alcohol, Lancet, 1948, 252,1001- 1004.
[14] Martensen-Larsen O. Treatment of alcoholism with a sensitising drug, Lancet, 1948, 252, 1004-1005

Over the next few years, there were several developments and discoveries. It emerged that the reaction with alcohol was due to a rapid increase in blood levels of acetaldehyde, a normal product of the first stage of alcohol metabolism but normally present in only small amounts before further metabolism. This increase was due to disulfiram's ability to inhibit the enzyme [acet]aldehyde dehydrogenase (ALDH) responsible for metabolising acetaldehyde to acetic acid and carbon dioxide. However, 50 years passed before it was realized that it was not disulfiram itself that caused ALDH inhibition but an active metabolite, S-methyl N,N-diethylthiolcarbamate sulfoxide.[15] Disulfiram is thus a *pro-drug* but whereas the usual minimum effective ALDH-inhibiting dose of disulfiram is around 200mg/day, the active metabolite is much more potent. Daily milligramme doses in single figures may be sufficient and this has important practical implications for the development of an effective 'disulfiram implant', as discussed in Ch.18 Like disulfiram, the active metabolite is readily absorbed through the skin – a fact that became apparent to US laboratory researchers who had handled the compound when they drank alcohol after work, just like their Danish counterparts in the mid 1940s.[16]

Disulfiram quickly attracted the attention of journalists and was hailed, in what is now a depressingly familiar pattern, as

---

[15] Ningaraj NS, Schloss JV, Williams TD, Faiman MD. Glutathione carbamoylation with S-methyl N,N-diethylthiolcarbamate sulfoxide and sulfone. Mitochondrial low Km aldehyde dehydrogenase inhibition and implications for its alcohol-deterrent action. Biochem Pharmacol. 1998; 55(6):749-56.
[16] Faiman M. Personal communication.

a 'wonder drug'. This was especially true in Denmark and Sweden, where, understandably, a certain amount of Nordic pride was activated. "Antabuse on its triumphant march throughout the world" was the headline in the Swedish newspaper *Dagen* in October, 1949.[17] As with any new drug, especially for a condition that was often difficult to treat, some physicians were equally enthusiastic and since the minimum effective dosage had not been established, they prescribed disulfiram on the principle – often dangerously attractive to patients as well as doctors – that large doses would be more effective than small ones. While 200-300mg/day is quite enough to produce a DAR for many patients, doses of ten times that amount were not uncommon in those early days and both severe side effects and severe DARs were noted.[18] A handful of patients died after being given needlessly large 'challenge doses' of alcohol to demonstrate the DAR, and a few clinicians may have given repeated alcohol challenges, either to reinforce the message or perhaps in the hope of setting up some kind of conditioned reflex that might associate the drinking of alcohol, in the mind of the patient, with unpleasant feelings. We don't think anyone has used disulfiram in this way since those early days and in our professional lifetimes, we have neither met nor heard of any clinician who did, but the myth that disulfiram is some kind of 'aversion therapy' persists in some quarters. It is discussed in more detail, and refuted, in Ch. 15. To set

---

[17] Kragh H. From disulfiram to Antabuse: the invention of a drug. Bull. Hist. Chem, 2008,33(2) 82-88
[18] Suh JJ, Pettinati HM, Kampman K, and O'Brien CP. The status of disulfiram a half of a century later. J Clin Psychopharmacol 2006:26;3, 290-302

these adverse events in historical context, recall that many citizens in those days were heavy smokers and had significant cardiac and pulmonary impairment. Even among people in their 30s and 40s, heart attacks were not rare and neither modern cardiac monitoring techniques nor cardiopulmonary resuscitation existed then. In the early days of lithium therapy for manic-depressive illness – also in the early 1950s – several deaths occurred from lithium toxicity before the correct dose-range was established and measuring blood lithium levels became simple and routine.

More level-headed physicians quickly pointed out that although disulfiram helped patients to achieve and maintain sobriety, many needed additional help. "It is important to emphasize that the chief value of Antabuse lies in the fact that it paves the way for psychotherapeutic procedures. ...Antabuse in conjunction with psychotherapy may prove superior to other methods of treatment of chronic alcoholism" [19] They also recognised that involving other people in supervising the consumption of disulfiram was important, once patients left hospital and were exposed again to the demands and temptations of even ordinary life. [20] Unfortunately, just as there are still many doctors (including psychiatrists) who think that what people who are 'depressed' need is 'antidepressant' medication and not much else, there was and is no shortage of physicians who took

---

[19] Barrera E, Osinski W, Davidoff E The use of Antabuse (Tetraethylthiuramdisulphide) in chronic alcoholics, Am J Psychiat 1950;107, 8-13
[20] Fox R. Antabuse as an adjunct to psychotherapy in alcoholism. *N Y J Med* 1958;58,1540-56.

much the same view of alcoholism and anti-alcoholism drugs. Fortunately, by the mid-1960s, there appeared the first study that showed how good results could be obtained even in the most unpromising patients by combining disulfiram, supervised administration and 'psychotherapeutic procedures'.[21] More on that study and its remarkable main author later.

---

[21] Bourne PG, Alford JA. Bowcock JZ. Treatment of skid-row alcoholics with Disulfiram Quart J Stud Alc 1966;27:42-.48.

Chapter 2. THE IMPORTANCE OF SUPERVISED CONSUMPTION. Family involvement, problem-oriented therapies and formal or informal treatment contracts.

Many alcoholics are very ambivalent about entering a period of abstinence, even when abstinence is clearly indicated. If they were not ambivalent, treatment would be much easier because they would either be 100% in favour of stopping drinking (in which case they would stop drinking and would unfailingly take disulfiram without supervision if it were prescribed) or they would be 100% against stopping (in which case, they would not be asking for treatment). It is therefore understandable that many of them are also ambivalent about taking disulfiram, because it so effectively stops them from doing what part of them still very much wants to do. This ambivalence is not, of course, unique to disulfiram. Compliance rates with many treatments are surprisingly low, even in life-endangering conditions like diabetes and hypertension. It is generally even worse for non-addictive psychotropic drugs like antidepressants and antipsychotics but good compliance is obviously of particular importance in alcoholics, precisely because their ambivalence is so marked. Indeed, for alcoholics, as with chronic schizophrenic patients, poor compliance with medication that is prescribed specifically to treat their condition is not just a common problem; it is a common and inherent characteristic of the condition that is being treated.

In the case of chronic schizophrenics, compliance with antipsychotic drugs can be improved by using depot injections. Because there is not yet a pharmacologically effective depot preparation of disulfiram (see Ch.18) other methods of improving compliance with oral medication have to be used. As with those too young, too old, too confused, too disorganised or too psychotic to take medicine reliably, or at all, these usually involve recruiting a third party. In hospital, nurses do the job. Outside hospital, family members or community nurses can take over. In the case of homeless patients with active tuberculosis, for whom prolonged and consistent treatment is essential, 'Directly Observed Treatment' programmes are now routine. For disulfiram, more imaginative arrangements may have to be made, involving people ranging from friends, neighbours and colleagues to probation officers and priests but it is important to emphasise that the arrangements are always a collaboration, not an imposition. The collaboration may be reluctant and ambivalent, especially at the start, but even probation-linked disulfiram (discussed later) involves the patient agreeing to collaborate with the courts and the probation service. That collaboration can, of course be withdrawn but the withdrawal will usually have obvious implications. This approach lends itself very well to both motivational interviewing [22] and the closely related community reinforcement model of treatment.[23]

Once somebody has accepted the role of supervisor, a little

---

[22] Miller WR. Motivational interviewing: research, practice, and puzzles. Addict Behav. 1996 Nov-Dec;21(6):835-42.

[23] Azrin NH, Sisson RW, Meyers R, Godley M. Alcoholism treatment by disulfiram and community reinforcement therapy. J Behav Ther Exp Psychiatry. 1982 Jun;13(2):105-12.

basic training is necessary. It sounds, and is, a simple enough procedure but as with many simple procedures, such as giving an intramuscular injection, measuring the blood pressure or taking the temperature with an oral thermometer, there are right and wrong ways of doing it and attention to detail is very important. Even in those studies where the importance of supervision is recognised, few spell out the process in detail. Azrin[24] is one of the exceptions and Table 1 gives his detailed but fundamentally simple advice:

Table 1. How to supervise disulfiram.

(a)	Identify a disulfiram monitor who would be substantially and negatively affected by resumption of drinking, e.g. spouse, family member, employer, lover, landlord.
(b)	The monitor should normally have regular, ideally daily, contact with the alcoholic.
(c)	Specify precisely the time and place where the disulfiram could be taken conveniently, with both persons present.
(d)	Have disulfiram taken at a time when other forms of medication are normally taken, i.e. the 'response-chaining' principle.
(e)	Grind up the disulfiram tablet and dissolve it in a drink (coffee, tea, juice) to avoid any suspicion of later expulsion.
(f)	If the monitor is not present when the patient has taken the disulfiram, the patient should take another tablet the same day, when the monitor is present, to provide absolute assurance to the monitor.

---

[24]Azrin NH.. Disulfiram and behaviour therapy: a social-biochemical model of alcohol abuse and treatment. In: Brewer C. (Ed.) Treatment Options in Addiction - Medical Management of Alcohol and Opiate Abuse. London. Gaskell - Royal College of Psychiatrists. 1993:19-28.

(g)	The patient should thank the monitor for taking the time to observe.
(h)	The monitor should comment on some positive attribute of the patient, that is associated with sobriety, i.e. job status, love by children, doing chores, financial security.
(i)	At each therapeutic session, the monitor attends with the patient, if possible, so that the therapist can instruct, supervise, and provide feedback to both.
(j)	At each therapeutic session, the disulfiram is taken in the presence of the therapist.
(k)	The monitor is to telephone the therapist if the patient omits taking disulfiram for three days; the therapist then telephones the patient to arrange a session.
(l)	When the usual 30-day supply of tablets is near-depleted, the monitor prompts and assists the patient to renew the prescription; failure to do so has been one of the most apparent major causes of discontinuing disulfiram.
(m)	The therapist asks the patient and monitor to rehearse probable situations which cause the reluctance to take the disulfiram, and teaches them how to overcome such interferences.
(n)	The patient is taught to view the use and ritual of taking disulfiram as a means of providing assurance to himself and his loved ones that he will not succumb to temptations that are otherwise beyond his control. It is emphasised that the central feature is the patient's desire, not coercion.

Merely offering someone a solution or suspension of disulfiram and watching while they swallow may not, unfortunately, be enough because unlike infants or the elderly, alcoholics are quite often tempted by their ambivalence to cheat. Those who agree to supervise disulfiram must, therefore, be aware of the tricks that patients sometime use to evade medication. Only one survey, covering 84 patients, seems to have studied them[25] but the list is a short one and perhaps surprisingly, most patients who try to evade disulfiram remain in treatment when their attempts are discovered and thwarted. The most important precaution is to make sure that the disulfiram is not only dissolved or suspended in water or yoghourt, as Azrin suggests but that it is also *seen to be swallowed*. That means that the patient should then drink a further glass of water or open his mouth to show that everything has been swallowed. However, there are ways of getting round even this protective ritual and it is not always the obvious suspects who are the devious ones. Here are the relevant tricks and proportions from that survey.

The commonest device – not so much cheating as testing-out - was to risk drinking in the hope that not much would happen. Of 20 patients who risked that, only half had a sufficiently deterrent DAR on doses of 200-300mg daily. That problem can usually be solved with a dose increase, though sometimes not without a brief admission to restore order and abstinence. The dosage issue is discussed in Ch. 9. Two patients induced vomiting to get rid of the disulfiram before it could be absorbed and four substituted tablets of a similar appearance – usually aspirin. (A variant of this technique, reported by an experienced US prescriber, was used by a patient who employed his skills as a die-maker to

---

[25] Brewer C. Patterns of compliance and evasion in treatment programmes which include supervised disulfiram. Alcohol Alc 1986;21:385-88

create fake tablets bearing the appropriate markings.) [26] Another ingenious patient – not included in the survey – carefully painted each tablet with transparent yacht varnish but his supervisor noticed the ruse. If vomiting is suspected, patients should remain within view for half an hour. Tablet substitution can be avoided by becoming familiar with any specific features of the disulfiram tablets, such as letters, numbers or a brand-name but also by the supervisor keeping control of the medication at all times. If – as very rarely happens – patients claim unconvincingly that nausea and vomiting prevent them from continuing disulfiram treatment, inviting them to distinguish between active and placebo medication in a single-blind trial will resolve the issue.[27]

Close family members often make good supervisors because they are often strongly motivated to help the patient. Becoming involved – and seeing the improvement that usually follows – also tends to make them feel better disposed to the patient and more optimistic. If supervision leads to conflicts and arguments, they can usually be resolved in therapist-led discussions involving the relevant family members and using a cognitive-behavioural 'couples therapy' approach.[28]

---

[26] McNichol R, Ewing J, Faiman M. Disulfiram (Antabuse) A unique medical aid to sobriety. Springfield. Charles Thomas. 1987, 10
[27] Ibid. 75
[28] Azrin N, Sissons R, Meyer SR, Godley M. Alcoholism treatment by disulfiram and community reinforcement therapy. J Behav Ther Exper Psychiat 1982;13, 105-112.

Fortunately, supervisors do not usually need to get into prolonged arguments with the patient if compliance is threatened or interrupted because the patient's implied or written therapeutic contract is with the doctor or other chief therapist and the job of persuading a vacillating patient ultimately falls to the professionals if the supervisor cannot do so. Just as important as the patient's agreement to accept supervision is the agreement that the supervisor can and must report promptly any failure or even delay in compliance. The fact that ALDH inhibition usually persists for several days after the last dose provides a unique cooling-off period before drinking can recommence, during which the supervisor and the treatment team have an opportunity to urge the patient to honour the agreement. However, we think Azrin's suggestion of not reporting failure of compliance unless it lasts for three days allows too long a period for ALDH inhibition to decline. 24 hours seems more appropriate. Those involved can also, of course, discuss the reasons that led to the cheating or refusal. No other alcoholism treatment has this built-in delay that acts as an early-warning system and can prevent an actual or potential lapse from becoming a relapse.

Motivating patients to accept a therapeutic contract including supervised disulfiram is no different in principle from motivating them to accept other therapeutic components about which patients may be – and often are – ambivalent. Phobic patients do not initially like graded exposure to feared objects or situations such as flying or spiders, and they could come to harm if exposure produces panic attacks. Drugs and surgery can have adverse effects. As with all medical, surgical, and psycho-social interventions, risks and benefits need to be discussed and choices need to be made but it is both common and legitimate for a clinician to encourage a patient to initiate and persevere with a mutually negotiated treatment plan and to adhere to informed and adequately considered therapeutic contracts.

Many alcoholics are still living in a family. Often, they are the husbands or partners of women for whom excessive drinking is a major problem of the relationship but not necessarily the only one. (Cognitive-) Behavioural Marital Therapy (BMT) or Couples Therapy is a widely-used evidence-based approach and can be easily adapted to include the taking of supervised disulfiram[29] as one of the changes to be made. There is good evidence that this specifically improves outcomes [30] though – as we note elsewhere – differences in the personality and 'style' of counsellors and psychotherapists may be more relevant to outcomes than the supposed theoretical basis of their interventions.

If patients are still working but estranged from their immediate family, someone at the workplace may be a suitable supervisor. Where the patient is the boss of the company or one of the directors, it may be possible to recruit a business partner or a secretary but some experimentation

---

[29] O'Farrell TJ, Bayog RD. Antabuse contracts for married alcoholics and their spouses: a method to maintain antabuse ingestion and decrease conflict about drinking. J Subst Abuse Treat. 1986;3(1):1-8.

[30] O'Farrell TJ, Choquette KA, Cutter HS. Couples relapse prevention sessions after behavioral marital therapy for male alcoholics: outcomes during the three years after starting treatment. J Stud Alcohol. 1998 Jul;59(4):357-70.

may be necessary before a satisfactory arrangement can be made. Even for patients who do not usually attend church, the local vicar or priest may be happy to help. (See Ch. 10 for an example) For patients with no family, or when years of alcoholic behaviour have alienated previously supportive family members or friends, then health professionals, hostel staff, or probation officers must substitute. (The kind of arrangement involving the local AA group described in Ch.15 is unfortunately, very uncommon.) Probation-linked disulfiram merits a separate discussion in Ch.10. A combined breathalyser and DSF breath monitor that can be attached to a mobile phone may facilitate supervision when work or location makes direct personal supervision difficult. [31] Disulfiram's prolonged action means that thrice or even twice weekly supervised dosing may provide adequate ALDH inhibition.

The frequent but brief patient-contacts needed in these more socially isolated patients are a key feature of the very successful OLITA programme (Outpatient Long-term Intensive Therapy for Alcoholics) developed in Germany and described in greater detail in Ch.11 . It combines supervised disulfiram with individually tailored management programmes targeting the patient's particular problems and situation as well as group support and meetings. However, it uses the same underlying principle of combining supervised disulfiram with appropriate problem-oriented interventions as

---

[31] Fletcher K. (2015) Disulfiram and the Zenalyser®: teaching an old dog new tricks. Alcohol Alcohol 50:255–6.

the individualised management that is more usual in general or private practice.

Chapter 3. THE MISLEADING 'RANDOMISED CONTROLLED TRIALS' OF DISULFIRAM

The importance of supervision was recognised by a few authors even in the early days of disulfiram treatment[32,33]. Numerous studies (discussed shortly) show that such third party involvement greatly improves compliance and therefore greatly improves the effectiveness of disulfiram. In 1986, an influential publication of the Royal College of Psychiatrists noted that "it is becoming more frequent for the doctor to suggest that a third person supervises the [disulfiram]...a relative or someone at work".[34]

However, as well as inhibiting ALDH, disulfiram seems to inhibit critical faculties in some reviewers of the literature. One prominent reviewer [35] dismissed disulfiram thus: "Disulfiram...lithium and various other substances have been tested in an attempt to increase abstinence rates in alcoholic patients, all with little or no success", though he seems to

---

[32] Fox R. Antabuse as an adjunct to psychotherapy in alcoholism. *N Y J Med* 1958;58:1540-1556.

[33] Billet SL. The use of Antabuse: An approach that minimises fear. Med Ann Dist Columb 1964;33:612-614

[34] Special Committee Of The Royal College Of Psychiatrists. Alcohol: our favourite drug. Tavistock Publications, London 1986

[35] Soyka M. Relapse prevention in alcoholism; recent advances and future possibilities. CNS Drugs 1997;4:313-327.

have changed his opinion recently.[36] The reference he gives for this statement (Fuller *et al* 1986)[37] is to a fairly classic randomised controlled trial (RCT). However, as briefly mentioned earler, disulfiram presents some unique difficulties in experimental design that do not apply to any other drug, apart from those with such obvious side-effects that blinding is impossible. One problem is that because the DAR is unpleasant and not entirely risk-free, some researchers (though not all) feel that it would be hazardous and unethical to inform the patients that half of them would be taking a placebo, since they might then be tempted to risk drinking with serious consequences. Fuller *et al*[37] got round this problem ingeniously. A third of the patients were prescribed 250mg of disulfiram daily, even though this dose would not have been enough to produce a sufficiently deterrent DAR in some patients (see Ch.9) A second group were told that they were receiving disulfiram but only had 1mg daily – a dose certainly far too small to produce a DAR but large enough to enable the researchers to persuade themselves that they were not, in fact, deceiving the patients. The remaining third received only the B-vitamin riboflavine.

Unfortunately, as was subsequently pointed out[38], although all patients were offered (and many received) follow-up counselling at weekly intervals for several months, in none of

---

[36] Mutschler J, Grosshans M, Soyka M, Rösner S. Current findings and mechanisms of action of difulfiram in the treatment of alcohol dependence. Pharmacopsychiat. 2016;49;1-5

[37] Fuller R, Branchey L, Brightwell D *et al*. Disulfiram treatment of alcoholism. JAMA 1986;256:1449-55.1986

[38] Brewer C. Disulfiram treatment for alcoholism. JAMA 1987;257:926.

these regular and labour-intensive therapeutic encounters was any attempt made to ensure that patients took at least one weekly supervised dose of disulfiram. The number of abstinent days increased slightly at 12 months in the group prescribed 250mg/day but the difference was clinically negligible. If common sense and some basic awareness of human nature had not sufficiently informed the researchers, the work of Azrin *et al*[39] had previously shown very clearly that patients prescribed disulfiram without third party supervision had nearly all discontinued it within three months. The small proportion of patients who regularly take disulfiram even without supervision – about 20% in the study by Fuller *et al* – were thus a very atypical and unusually compliant group of patients. They may have been similar to the patients in the 'treatment vs advice' study by Edwards *et al*,[40] nearly half of whom had good or improved outcomes at 12 months despite having no active treatment following an elaborate initial research-oriented assessment. (See Ch.5 for a more detailed discussion.) It is probable that the cooperative 20% of Fuller *et al's* patients, and their counterparts in other studies, simply demonstrated the 'healthy complier effect' – an important aspect of placebo and non-specific effects discussed more thoroughly in Ch.7.

---

[39] Azrin NH, Sissons RW, Meyer RJ, & Godley M. Alcoholism treatment by disulfiram and community reinforcement therapy. J Behav Ther Exp Psychiat 1982;13:105-12.

[40] Edwards G, Orford J, Egert S et al. Alcoholism: a controlled trial of 'treatment' and 'advice'. Quarterly J Stud Alc 1977;38:1004-33.

A much bigger problem is that even if patients in a RCT do not know whether they are receiving disulfiram or a placebo, the deterrent effect tends to work just as well in the placebo group as in the active one because both groups are equally reluctant to run the risk of a DAR. As mentioned, exactly the same principle applies to speed cameras. All motorists know that some speed cameras may be faulty or even inactive 'placebo' cameras (which are much cheaper to install and maintain than the real thing) but unless drivers know for sure which ones are real and which ones are not, they nearly all behave as if every camera were active and they moderate their speed accordingly. Average speed cameras, which can monitor and record the speed of an individual car over several miles of road, have an even greater deterrent effect. This should have been rather obvious to any researcher who thought about how disulfiram works but it was not until Marilyn Skinner, an American psychologist working in Paris, published a meta-analysis, which made this important point very clear,[41] that it gained a prominent place in the evidence-base. The nature of disulfiram means that classic, 'gold-standard' blinded trials are not appropriate but this is also true of comparisons between medical and surgical treatments. It does not mean that fair comparisons are impossible.

In subsequent published correspondence, Fuller accepted the importance of supervision and reported that he had attempted, unsuccessfully, to get funding for a further study in which the contribution of adequate disulfiram supervision

---

[41] Skinner, MD, Lahmek P, Pham H, Aubin HJ. Disulfiram efficacy in the treatment of alcohol dependence: a meta analysis. Plos One 2014, 9(2): e87366

would be separately assessed. [42] He also noted that unsupervised disulfiram was the usual practice in the US, which was clearly true at the time though equally clearly, US clinicians like Azrin and several others recognised the importance of supervision. As so often happens after the publication of influential papers, subsequent criticism, published merely as letters in the journal's correspondence pages, is often ignored by later reviewers, even if it is accurate[43].

Although the study by Fuller *et al* naturally attracts the attention of the reviewers because of its apparently impeccable design, its limitations, acknowledged by Fuller himself, should have served as a warning to reviewers who failed to distinguish between the many trials of *unsupervised* disulfiram, which are mainly negative and often rather badly designed, and the much smaller number of trials in which the consumption of disulfiram is more or less diligently supervised. It is interesting that the main authors of these supervised trials are often psychologists, rather than physicians or psychiatrists. The study by Azrin *et al*, giving the most positive results of all such trials, was singled out by Saunders[44] as having a particularly convincing experimental

---

[42] Fuller R. Disulfiram treatment of alcoholism (letter) JAMA1987;257:927

[43] Bhopal R, Tonks A. The role of letters in reviewing research (Editorial) BMJ 1994;308:158-223

[44] Saunders B. Treatment does not work: some criteria of failure. In: The misuse of alcohol: crucial issues in dependence, treatment and prevention. Heather N, Robertson I, Davies P (Eds): London: Croom Helm 1985:102-116.

design, even though Saunders, a psychologist, gave very little prominence or credit to the inclusion of disulfiram. Marilyn Skinner, the principal author of the important and most recent meta-analysis, is also a psychologist. Unlike all the other drugs used or recommended for alcoholism, encouragement to use disulfiram and much of the research that justifies that encouragement has originated not with physicians or drug companies but with clinical psychologists using cognitive-behavioural approaches who saw clearly and at first hand how disulfiram improved their results and could be easily and rationally integrated into their practice. Clinical psychologists and counsellors who use evidence-based interventions (and their accountants) can relax once they find a prescribing physician to work with. The 'disulfiram revival'[45] definitely does not represent a take-over bid by doctors!

William Miller, another psychologist and a respected reviewer of the alcoholism effectiveness literature, classified alcoholism treatment into those for which sound evidence for effectiveness exists; those whose effectiveness or specific effectiveness has yet to be demonstrated; and those which are demonstrably lacking in any specific effect. At one time he placed disulfiram firmly in the latter category[46] but around

---

[45] Grover S, Basu D. The revival (or, rather, survival) of disulfiram. Addiction. 2004 Jun;99(6):785.

[46] Miller WR, Hester RK. The effectiveness of alcoholism treatment methods: what research reveals. In: Treating addictive behaviours: Processes of change. Miller, W. R., Heather, N .(Eds). New York: Plenum. 1986.

1990, he changed his opinion and now regards supervised (but not unsupervised) disulfiram as a treatment of proven effectiveness [47] In recent meta-analyses of the literature, two of the psycho-social treatment approaches that consistently come out well are Community Reinforcement Therapy (CRT) and Behavioural Marital Therapy, both of which lend themselves to (and often incorporate) supervised disulfiram, as already mentioned.[48,49,50,51]

---

[47] Miller WR. The effectiveness of alcoholism treatment modalities: causes and consequences of alcohol abuse. Hearings before the committee on governmental affairs, part III: US Senate. 1989:171-185

[48] Holder H, Longabaugh R, Miller W, Rubonis,A. The cost effectiveness of treatment for alcoholism: a first approximation. . J Stud Alc. 1991;52:517-540

[49] Finney JW, Monahan SC. The cost-effectiveness of treatment for alcoholism: a second approximation. J Stud Alc. 1996;57:229-243.

[50] O'Farrell TJ, Bayog RD. Antabuse contracts for married alcoholics and their spouses: a method to maintain antabuse ingestion and decrease conflict about drinking. J Subst Abuse Treat1986;3:11-8.

[51] O'Farrell TJ. Treating alcohol problems: marital and family interventions. Guilford Press, New York 1993.

Chapter 4. THE JAPANESE CONNECTION

If you were told about an easily identifiable, non-Islamic group of adults in whom alcoholism was virtually unknown, rather than unusual or relatively uncommon, you would probably assume that they were a small, clinically irrelevant group who all shared a culture or religion that had social mechanisms for enforcing abstinence or moderation. Perhaps a community like the Amish of New England. You would probably say, rightly, that the existence of such groups tells us nothing that helps us to treat the alcoholics who knock on our clinic doors, because we cannot turn them into devout Amish even if we wanted to. Only anthropological readers might register a flicker of interest but there is one such group in whom the absence of heavy drinking is not explained by cultural factors and we can learn a lot from them about ways of improving treatment - and about disulfiram. This group consists of all the people in Japan (and in some of its neighbours) who are homozygous[52] for a gene that gives them a very inefficient version of ALDH. They number about 8% of the Japanese population, so there are about nine million of them in a country where alcohol use is long established and normal.

Aldehyde dehydrogenase (ALDH) is not a single enzyme. As with many other enzymes, most people harbour several sub-types, labelled variously ALDH1, ALDH1A1, ALDH2, ALDH2*1, and ALDH2*2, among others. The proportions of

---

[52] Note for the unmedical. 'Homozygous' means inheriting a gene from both parents.

these sub-types are genetically determined and also vary between different organs but the liver is probably the most important site for alcohol metabolism. Some ALDH sub-types, notably ALDH2*2, are much less efficient at metabolising acetaldehyde than the average and people who inherit mainly 'inefficient' ALDH therefore get high acetaldehyde levels and experience the equivalent of a DAR if they drink more than very small amounts of alcohol. In American, European, Central Asian and Pacific Island populations, only a tiny percentage of people have such predominantly inefficient ALDH sub-types. In contrast, approximately a third of East Asians (Japanese, Chinese, and Koreans) show a characteristic response to drinking alcohol, due to predominance of ALDH2 sub-types. The proportion increases with increasing longitude, reaching around 50% in Japan. For many of that 50%, the reaction with alcohol is not so severe that it makes drinking almost intolerable. Many Chinese, Koreans and Japanese get what the scientific literature still calls an 'Oriental flush' when they drink, but it does not necessarily stop them from drinking normal social amounts or even quite a lot more. However, many heterozygotes[53] drink little or no alcohol and the incidence of alcoholism among them is about half the normal Japanese figure. (See below)

These 'flushers' have usually inherited inefficient ALDH from only one parent and are thus heterozygous for the inefficient sub-type. They have a mixture of efficient ALDH2*1 and inefficient ALDH2*2 (genotypically represented as ALDH2*1/*2) and their reaction to alcohol is

---

[53] Inheriting from only one parent.

similar to that experienced by patients taking an inadequate dose of disulfiram. In contrast, about 10% of Japanese inherit inefficient ALDH2*2 from both parents (genotype ALDH2*2/*2). When they sip their first glass of saké or the up-market whiskies that are popular with Japanese 'salarymen', these homozygotes soon discover that anything more than a small sip makes them feel increasingly unwell and the effectiveness of disulfiram would not surprise them. Japanese homozygotes experience the lifelong and unavoidable effects of Nature's version of supervised disulfiram at adequate dose levels. Since most of them are, in other respects, average, 'normal' Japanese citizens, that means that most of them would otherwise grow up to become typical Japanese users and sometimes abusers of alcohol in a country where most people drink alcohol, yet both social drinking and alcoholism are vanishingly rare among them.[54] Opinions differ slightly about the precise degree of rarity but not about the rarity itself. In a survey of 655 Japanese alcoholics and 461 controls, Higuchi concluded, "The [ALDH2*2/*2] genotype was found in none of the alcoholics, suggesting that individuals with homozygous [ALDH2*2] never become alcoholics". [55] Chen *et al.* qualified this view only very slightly. "The gene status of ALDH2*2/*2 alone can give very considerable but not - as previously thought - complete protection against the

---

[54] Sun F, Tsuritani I, Yamada Y. (2002) Contribution of genetic polymorphisms in ethanol-metabolizing enzymes to problem drinking behavior in middle-aged Japanese men. Behav Genet 32:229–36.
[55] Higuchi S. (1994) Polymorphisms of ethanol metabolizing enzyme genes and alcoholism. Alcohol Alcohol Suppl 2:29–34.

development of alcohol dependence". [56] Normally, cells contain both ALDH1 and ALDH2 subtypes and ALDH2, in particular, is found in both the cytosole (the intracellular fluid) and the mitochondria. The mitochondrial form is the more efficient but in homozygotes, mitochondrial ALDH2 is absent.

The simple and obvious explanation for the virtual absence of alcoholism among ALDH2*2/*2 homozygotes is that alcohol in more than minimal quantities (such as might be contained in a sauce, for example) causes an unpleasant reaction that is virtually identical to the DAR that accounts for disulfiram's deterrent (and thus therapeutic) effect.[57] The extremely rare reported exceptions among homozygous patients typically involve homozygous individuals who also have severe anxiety or other forms of psychological distress and try to use alcohol to drown their discomforts despite the unpleasant consequences, but such patients never manage to drink more than relatively modest amounts of alcohol spread over 24 hours. They sip alcohol steadily rather than gulping it. It is also possible that other genetic factors enable those exceptional ALDH2*2/*2 homozygotes to tolerate these levels of alcohol consumption. For example, less efficient variants of alcohol dehydrogenase (ADH) could cause slower alcohol metabolism at the first stage of alcohol breakdown and thus reduce the level of acetaldehyde production. (See

---

[56] Chen Y-C, Lu R-B, Peng G-S, et al. (1999) Alcohol metabolism and cardio vascular response in an alcoholic patient homozygous for the ALDH2*2 variant gene allele. Alc Clin Exp Res 23:1853–60.

[57] A presumably heterozygotic Japanese friend told me that the flushing phenomenon was never discussed when he was at school. It is – or was – something that Japanese adolescents just discover for themselves.

also Ch.19.) Genetically and/or psychologically determined differences in cardiovascular responses or tolerance of discomfort might also play a part. Nevertheless, in large Japanese surveys such as those cited above, the incidence of alcoholism in homozygotes is zero or close to zero.

In the study referenced above, Sun et al. also found that in those who are heterozygous for inefficient ALDH, the incidence of alcoholism was around 5% compared with around 10% in those with 'efficient' or 'western-style' ALDH. This represents a clear dose-response in terms of ALDH inhibition and also strongly suggests that ALDH inhibition rather than any direct neurophysiological action of disulfiram is the crucial pharmacological component of its effectiveness. Similarly, Bickel et al.[58] and Newton-Howes et al.[59] document the fact that if patients continue drinking on standard doses of DSF, raising the dose will usually secure abstinence. The issue of dosage is discussed in greater detail in Ch.9 Although almost all researchers agree that the deterrent effect of the DAR is the only important pharmacological effect of disulfiram in alcoholism, a few authors have suggested that its ability to inhibit other enzymes, notably dopamine-beta-hydroxylase, might have anti-craving effects.[60] Given that patients in double-blind

---

[58] Bickel WK, Rizzuto P, Zielony RD, Klobas J, Pangiosonlis P, Mernit R, Knight WF. Combined Behavioral and Pharmacological Treatment of Alcoholic Methadone Patients. J Subst Abuse. 1988-1989;1(2):161-71.

[59] Newton-Howes G, Levack WM, McBride S, Gilmor M, Tester R. Non-physiological mechanisms influencing disulfiram treatment of alcohol use disorder: A grounded theory study. Drug Alc Depend 2016;165:126-31.

[60] Mutschler J, Bühler M, Grosshans M, Diehl A, Mann K, Kiefer F. Disulfiram, an option for the treatment of pathological gambling? Alcohol Alcohol. 2010 Mar-Apr;45(2):214-6.

trials receiving placebo disulfiram appear to be equally deterred from drinking, that hypothesis seems unlikely or at best of marginal relevance. (I first discussed the Japanese connection in detail in: Brewer C. Supervised disulfiram is more effective in alcoholism than naltrexone or acamprosate - or even psychotherapy. How it works and why it matters. Adicciones. 2005. 17(4); 285-96. from which parts of this chapter are taken).

Chapter 5. THE VARIETIES OF ALCOHOLIC EXPERIENCE

From the clinician's point of view, alcoholic patients – like all patients – fall into two broad categories: easy patients and difficult or challenging patients. They also, of course, exist on a spectrum but a surprising proportion of alcoholic patients inhabit the easier end of the spectrum. There is good evidence that for a significant proportion of alcohol abusers, once they accept that they have a problem, stopping or reducing drinking is often achieved with little effort and with little or no professional help. One of the few really important British practical contributions to alcoholism treatment research – briefly mentioned earlier - is the 1977 study by Griffith Edwards and his team that compared 'treatment' with 'advice'.[61] This study seems to be unknown (or is possibly suppressed) in the 'celebrity rehab' clinics and chains that routinely tell any alcoholics thinking of changing their habits that unless they admit themselves immediately, and preferably stay for at least 28 days, they will undoubtedly die soon and horribly. The truth, as the British study showed, is much more encouraging. One hundred married, male alcoholics seeking treatment for the first time had a single, very thorough research-style assessment interview and were then randomised to two groups. The 'treatment' group were offered whichever of the conventional treatments of the period was thought most

---

[61] Edwards G, Orford J, Egert S et al. Alcoholism: a controlled trial of 'treatment' and 'advice'. Quart J Stud Alc 1977;38:1004-33.

appropriate. The 'advice' group (and their wives) were told, in effect: 'The most important thing is that you have accepted that you have a problem, so try at least to drink a lot less or better still, stop altogether. Our research team will visit or telephone both of you once a month during the next year to see how you're doing but it really depends on you and your wife. Good luck!'

The results a year later were interesting in two respects. Firstly, there were no statistically significant differences in outcome between the two groups, though there were some interesting non-significant ones. For example, the 'treatment' group averaged 84 days off work in the following 12 months for sickness or unemployment, vs 63 days for the 'advice' group, despite 50% more AA attendance. Ten 'treatment' patients spent more than 8 weeks in hospital during the year (including six who stayed more than 12 weeks) vs none in the 'advice' group. Secondly, in both groups, about 40-50% (depending on who was asked) had improved, including around 20% who had stopped drinking. The proportions of those who were unchanged, drank less but still had some problems, or drank even more, were similar in both groups. These outcomes are similar to the considerable improvement reported by many patients in RCTs of psychotherapy, following a single interview aimed at assessment rather than treatment.[62] When it comes to planning alcoholism treatment, it is surely very significant that patients in both groups rated their initial interview and advice as one of the four most

---

[62] Sloane R, Staples F, Cristol A, Yorkston N, Whipple K. Psychotherapy versus Behaviour Therapy. Cambridge, MA. Harvard University Press. 1975, passim

important factors in their improvement and by far the most important aspect of their treatment experience – well above the contributions of AA or of any out-patient or in-patient intervention, thus confirming that 'easy' patients tend to do well whatever treatment, and however much or little of it, they receive. The mechanisms underlying these large and lasting improvements with minimal professional input have much in common with the placebo and non-specific effects of alcoholism treatment discussed in Ch. 7.

Here is a case history of one of those 'easy' patients. Karl was born in Germany but lived in London with two children and his English wife and he was in his late 50s when I first saw him. By that time, he had acquired an international reputation as a technical consultant in theatre and TV productions and his work took him all over the world. There was some alcoholism in his family background but not much and Karl himself had been an essentially unproblematic social drinker until his 40s. Unfortunately, the increasing international travel that went with his increasing reputation meant more and more lonely nights in foreign hotels, often preceded by well-oiled dinners with his grateful clients.

Drink eased his loneliness but came at the cost of increasing physical dependence on alcohol and ill health. Eventually, he sought help from his GP, who referred him for treatment. By this time, he was drinking a bottle of spirits a day and had developed classic alcoholic morning drinking to ward off classic alcoholic withdrawal symptoms. He looked unwell and his liver was enlarged, with significantly disturbed liver function tests (LFTs). Previous unaided attempts at stopping drinking had failed because of the severity of his withdrawal symptoms and since he wanted to get back to work as soon as possible – a common situation with self-employed professionals – it seemed best to admit him to hospital for withdrawal, rather than try (and possibly fail) to do so as an out-patient.

Withdrawal was not difficult and he was fit for discharge after five days. The problem then was how best to keep him dry when he resumed his punishing schedule. He was unwilling to cancel any of his impending commitments, in part because he seemed to be one of the top people in his field and didn't want to let his clients down. Although detailed discussion of his subsequent treatment was deferred until he had sobered up, it had already been suggested that while supervised disulfiram was one of the options, directly supervising disulfiram would be difficult unless his wife travelled with him when he was out of the country. That wasn't really practicable but he could try taking it 'over the phone', as it were, so that she could hear him crunching the tablets and ostentatiously swallowing them. (This was well before mobile phones enabled a degree of distant real-time monitoring of compliance.) If that didn't work, we would have to arrange for his clients to do the supervising – a much less desirable alternative.

In the event, the system worked well but it became clear that he was probably an 'easy' patient because of something that happened at his first follow-up appointment a few days after discharge. Soon after he sat down, he took out a letter he had written on his own initiative to all his friends and colleagues. It read something like this:

'Dear... I have come to realise that I have developed a serious alcohol problem and that I must stop drinking completely and permanently. It may not have affected my work much but it has certainly damaged my health and affected my family life. I am having treatment for the problem but I am writing this to make it clear that from now on, you must never offer me alcohol or try to persuade me to join you in drinking it.'

This was such a spontaneous, unusual and public statement of his commitment to sobriety that I felt immediately that his risk of relapse was low, and so it turned out. Karl took disulfiram consistently for six months. During that time, his travels made face-to-face follow up infrequent but we did some of it by telephone. Within a few weeks, his LFTs returned to normal and stayed that way, and he stopped looking unwell. By the time we agreed to try without the disulfiram after six months, he seemed to have adapted very well to an alcohol-free existence and there were really no problems for which counselling – let alone formal psychotherapy – was indicated. He never suggested controlled drinking as a later treatment goal (See Ch. 12). It was agreed that he and/or his wife would contact me if there were any concerns but they never did. Except that every Christmas for several years thereafter, they sent a card confirming that he was remaining sober and that life was good.

At the other end of the 'easiness' spectrum, we need not concern ourselves here with those patients whose extreme reluctance to change is reflected in their refusal to have even an initial specialist consultation. They do not merit serious therapeutic attention (as opposed to attempts at health education) unless and until they become much less ambivalent, although we may be able to teach their families or employers effective ways of bringing them into treatment.[63] If they get as far as a specialist service and cooperate with conventional psychosocial treatments like counselling or AA attendance but do not improve, disulfiram can be very useful not just for treating them but also for assessing their real level of commitment. That common situation is discussed in Ch. 6.

Both cost-effectiveness (in state-funded programmes) and proper professional ethics (in private ones) should mean that 'easy' patients ought not to be required to have more treatment than they need. In public services, that allows more resources to be directed at those who, though willing in principle to cooperate with treatment and to learn new habits of thinking and behaving, find - sometimes to their genuine surprise and annoyance - that the old habits continue to assert themselves. This group demonstrate their stated willingness to change by regular attendance at clinics or AA groups. If advised to have counselling, psychotherapy or assertiveness training, or to take medication such as acamprosate or naltrexone, they do so, but they keep on relapsing, often to

---

[63] Sisson R, Azrin N. Family member involvement to initiate and promote treatment of problem drinkers. J Behav Ther Exper Psychiat 1986;17, 15-21.

the despair of themselves and their helpers. As also discussed in Ch. 6, Sereny et al. described 73 such patients with three or more relapses despite adhering to a comprehensive conventional treatment programme.[64] When this happens, there is a tendency to blame the patient and 'poor motivation', but if the patients are doing all that is asked, is there not perhaps a case for blaming (or at least examining) the methods used to teach them new habits? In these cases, we should surely concentrate on the most efficient methods of relapse prevention, especially at the start of treatment when relapse may undermine the patient's fragile belief in his ability to change.

Patients entering treatment for the first time are an unknown quantity. Many, it is clear will turn out to be 'easy' and time will soon tell which of them will be 'difficult' but with patients who have had previous treatment, their place on that important spectrum will already have become increasingly clear. The patient who last attended a couple of years ago after successful treatment and has now returned after just a few weeks of excessive drinking is probably still relatively 'easy' and likely to cooperate with treatment again. Conversely, the patient who is back in the ward or the out-patient clinic (or the cells) a few months or even a few weeks or days after a previous episode of treatment characterised by poor cooperation and unhappy staff-patient relationships, is clearly one of the 'difficult'. Adding disulfiram can make life

---

[64] Sereny G, Sharma V, Holt J, Gordis E. Mandatory supervised Antabuse therapy in an out-patient alcoholism program: a study. Alc Clin Exper Res 1986;10:290-292.

easier for many of these unfortunate patients and their clinicians but even supervised disulfiram patients can remain difficult. Here is an example.

James was 25 when I first saw him and he was not new to alcoholism treatment. Several previous admissions to private 12-step clinics, for whom disulfiram was anathema, had been followed by early relapse and his family were running out of money as well as patience. He worked in the small family business and he was hoping to get married. His was clearly a case for disulfiram and he agreed to take it. Although he drank heavily, he had only mild withdrawal symptoms but had to be admitted overnight before he stopped drinking for long enough to start taking 200mg of disulfiram daily. He still lived with his parents and they supervised the disulfiram diligently but after a few weeks, James tried drinking and got very little reaction. After another overnight admission, he started on 400mg, which he tolerated well. This kept him dry for several months but when he again tried drinking, the reaction was still unimpressive. It was expected that he would try drinking even after the dose was increased to 600mg, and he did but this time, the reaction was quite severe. He did not repeat the experiment but he tried several times to evade treatment, usually after several months of abstinence had made his parents lower their guard. Although he did marry, and abstained for much of the next several years,[65] the marriage eventually broke down and in the consequent absence of efficient supervision (and adequate

---

[65] Brewer C. Long-term, high-dose disulfiram in the treatment of alcohol abuse. Brit J Psychiat 1993;163:687-689

motivation) he resumed heavy drinking.

DURATION OF TREATMENT

Long term outcome studies are notoriously difficult and expensive to do. They are often vitiated by high drop-out rates and this is true of all treatment modalities. However, Fuller et al[66] lost a valuable opportunity to use a well-funded 12-month RCT to study supervised disulfiram because they chose not to supervise it. Azrin followed up a small cohort for 2 years but the undeserved unpopularity of supervised disulfiram has generally excluded it from large trials such as Project MATCH. (See Ch. 17) Galanter, whose 'network therapy' makes extensive use of disulfiram, supervised by a network of family members, friends or colleagues, feels that 12 months is a reasonable minimum.[67] He finds that abstinence is often "well established" by then but he accepts that some patients wish (or should be advised) to take it for longer. As well as patients like James, there are several case reports of patients who evidently felt they needed the protection of disulfiram for 10 or 15 years. At least two of these involved supervised disulfiram[68]. A patient of one of the authors of the 1987 textbook ("a university professor") had been taking it for 17 years.[69] Conversely, one comes

---

[66] Fuller et al 1986 *op.cit.*
[67] Galanter M. Network therapy for alcohol and drug abuse. London. Guilford. 1999.
[68] Brewer C. Using disulfiram to maintain controlled drinking: A case report with a 14-year follow-up. Addiction Res 1996;3:231-235
[69] McNichol R, Ewing J, Faiman M. Disulfiram (Antabuse) A unique medical aid to sobriety. Springfield. Charles Thomas. 1987, 12

across patients – like Karl, the theatre technician - who seem to remain abstinent or achieve controlled drinking for many years after only a few months of supervised disulfiram but courses of less than six months are likely to be too short for most patients.

The highly important German OLITA study, (discussed in more detail in Ch. 11) strongly suggests that for the undoubtedly 'difficult' and rather challenging patients that formed their cohort, somewhere between 18 and 24 months of supervised disulfiram is advisable for the best outcome. We agree with Galanter that where disulfiram is indicated, 12 months is a desirable minimum for patients who are reasonably well integrated with work and domestic life. If patients are reluctant to commit to such a long period, one can suggest they try it for 6 months and then review the situation. If, as is common, six months of abstinence is the longest they have ever experienced since adolescence, they may well have got used to the experience by then and be willing to continue it. The question of graduating from abstinence to experiments with controlled drinking is discussed in Ch. 12.

Chapter 6. DISULFIRAM'S ROLE IN RETAINING AMBIVALENT PATIENTS IN TREATMENT AND IDENTIFYING THE UNMOTIVATED

All experienced clinicians are familiar with patients at the extreme end of the ambivalence spectrum. We see them in the medical or surgical wards when they are admitted for alcohol-related injuries or illnesses.[70] It is clear that they are drinking not just a bit too much but far too much and if they are visited by their long-suffering families, the extent and acute danger of their alcohol problem may become even more clear to us. Unfortunately, any requests for them to be seen by a psychiatrist or alcoholism specialist are made by the admitting physicians or surgeons and not by the patients, who either do not accept that they have a really serious alcohol problem or do accept it but decline to have any treatment. They will probably cut down on their drinking for a few weeks while their damaged organs recover, or their fractures heal, but they will soon be drinking heavily again

---

[70] Note for the unmedical: Apart from several cancers that are clearly related to alcoholism, and a very significant proportion of domestic, industrial and traffic accidents and injuries, the main medical complications include cirrhosis of the liver, acute and chronic pancreatitis, hypertension, heart disease, strokes, cerebral atrophy, dementia, neuropathy, epilepsy and diabetes. Even when not lethal, they can be very disabling. In Korsakov's syndrome, there is total and usually permanent loss of recent memory. Alcoholics with cirrhosis can die slowly of liver failure but also of torrential bleeding from internal varicose veins that can cause death in minutes. When alcoholism undermines general health, even normally treatable conditions like pneumonia can prove fatal, as can alcohol withdrawal.

with their equally alcoholic friends or on their own, according to habit and circumstances. If they later agree to an out-patient consultation, they will do so reluctantly and may cancel the appointment on the day.

This sort of patient cannot easily be persuaded to accept treatment but there are moderately encouraging studies[71] that indicate how families can be given training in techniques for putting pressure on alcoholic members in ways that increase the likelihood of their accepting treatment. They are more effective (or less ineffective) than the confrontational techniques recommended in some 12-step clinics, although the details are beyond the scope of this book. When and if the patient changes his mind about treatment, we can welcome him to the clinic. Offering to consider a controlled drinking approach, perhaps with the help of naltrexone, may make it easier for him to accept treatment, on the understanding that the failure rate is high and that the only alternative is abstinence for at least a few months, almost certainly needing disulfiram to succeed.

Another sort of ambivalent patient seems to have no fundamental objection to accepting that he has an alcohol problem or that it needs treatment. He may be willing to give both his protesting organs and his alcohol-related work and family problems a rest at a residential rehab. Typically after admission, he regularly attends the numerous groups and one-to-one therapy sessions that fill the rehab's working day

---

[71] Sisson R, Azrin N. Family member involvement to initiate and promote treatment of problem drinkers. J Behav Ther Exper Psychiat 1986;17, 15-21.

and he may even make some useful contributions in groups but when he leaves the clinic after the customary 28 days, it is not long before he resumes drinking. When you see him again in the outpatient department or in your consulting room, he is full of apparently sincere regret at his inability to remain abstinent, despite continued attendance, in some cases, at his local AA group. In some countries, and in some types of employment, his apparent willingness to cooperate repeatedly with manifestly ineffective treatment may be related to the generosity or otherwise of the arrangements for sick-leave, retirement on medical grounds and payment for alcoholism treatment.

If naltrexone or acamprosate haven't already been prescribed, this sort of patient will probably agree to take them but whether or not he actually does so is another matter. Oral naltrexone is hardly ever given under supervision in alcoholism treatment (in contrast to its use for opiate dependence, where supervision is a crucial feature of some probation-linked programmes and a few ordinary ones). Its effectiveness in very ambivalent alcoholic patients has not been evaluated and in any case, even in countries where controlled drinking appears on the treatment menu, this patient would not be a promising candidate. Acamprosate is even less likely to work and the thrice-daily dosage schedule makes supervision impracticable. (The marginal effectiveness of both these drugs compared with disulfiram is documented in Ch. 17.) Some of these patients may even quietly enjoy telling the prescriber that they have been taking the medication but it doesn't seem to be working.

Suggesting disulfiram in this situation typically produces some interesting responses. The patient may immediately refuse to take it but that involves a public declaration to any interested parties that he doesn't really want to deal with his drink problem. Since many of these patients are already under serious pressure from family or employers, that is a dangerous position to maintain and few do so. Because those few are clearly not interested in treatment, there is no point in further clinic attendance unless and until they change their minds and agree to take disulfiram under supervision. Indeed, making this stipulation can be diagnostic as well as therapeutic, because it quickly identifies both the totally unmotivated, who at that stage are clearly unsuitable for any treatment, and the rather less ambivalent, whose motivation may yet be engaged and strengthened. If they can be persuaded to at least start taking disulfiram under what obviously needs to be especially rigorous supervision and with dose increases and alcohol challenges if necessary, then some of them may stay on it – and thus remain abstinent – for long enough for other components of treatment to have a chance of changing their attitudes to drinking in the medium and longer term. In the first few weeks and months of treatment, lapses (refusal to take disulfiram for a day or two but resuming it before heavy drinking – or any drinking – occurs) or even brief relapses (refusing disulfiram for long enough to drink heavily, but willing, if necessary, to accept a brief admission to start disulfiram again) do not always predict the failure of treatment. As the OLITA study demonstrates, dogged but kindly persistence by the treatment team, together with family and other social support, can retain a useful proportion of these patients in treatment and enable them eventually to benefit from specific psychotherapeutic and employment-promoting interventions.

I was once asked to see an alcoholic in his early thirties who had been treated in most of Britain's fashionable and expensive rehabs and drying-out establishments without any lasting benefit. The problems started when he inherited a lot of money while at art school[72] and quickly went to the bad. Whenever he was admitted, he was usually a model patient but he never abstained for more than a week or two after discharge. Eventually, someone suggested that he should try disulfiram and an appointment was made – and kept. He came with his parents, who were naturally rather worried about him. I went through the history and he agreed that he had not managed to abstain for long in the real world despite much conventional but non-pharmacological treatment, so I suggested that it was time for a trial of disulfiram. I didn't have to explain how it worked because like most experienced alcoholic patients, he already knew.

He agreed immediately. I then explained that because of the regrettable but very understandable tendency of patients not to take disulfiram regularly, it was vital to take it under supervision. Since he lived quite near his parents, the obvious arrangement was for him to go to their house, or vice versa, three times a week.

After hesitating for a few seconds, he agreed to this. Finally, I told him that as an added precaution, the disulfiram tablets had to be dissolved in water before being swallowed because,

---

[72] Such patients are known in the trade as 'trustafarians'.

equally regrettably and understandably, some patients only *pretended* to swallow them and then spat them out at the first opportunity. He thought for a while, then gave a friendly grin. 'I can see what you're trying to do, doctor', he said. 'You're trying to get me to stop drinking, aren't you. Well, I'm not going to do it.'

Chapter 7. COMPONENTS OF EFFECTIVENESS IN DISULFIRAM TREATMENT AND OTHER INTERVENTIONS FOR ALCOHOLISM – including placebo and non-specific effects

All evidence-based treatments – pharmacological, psychological and surgical - have non-specific or placebo effects as well as specific effects and disulfiram is no exception. The powerful deterrent effect, in some cases, of implants of disulfiram which actually have no measurable pharmacological activity (already mentioned, and discussed in more detail in Ch. 18) underlines the importance of three separate but mutually reinforcing factors that are unique features of treatment with ALDH-inhibiting drugs.

Firstly, there is the real and unpleasant DAR. Patients taking disulfiram may know at various levels about this reaction. All of them will have been warned about it and many will believe what they are told without testing it out for themselves. Some know of it vicariously from observing or hearing about the reaction in other alcoholics. A variable proportion of sceptical or foolish patients make the discovery for themselves by actual experiment. It is only because disulfiram has, and is known to have, this very real likelihood of an unpleasant interaction with alcohol that it deters many patients from drinking by the mere fact of taking it. Further evidence for a specific deterrent effect of the DAR comes from the Japanese studies already discussed.

Secondly, taking disulfiram regularly surely has certain symbolic connotations. It tells us that here is a patient who is willing, however uncertainly or ambivalently, to surrender some control over his freedom or urge to drink. Such a patient announces both to himself and to the wider world that he is not merely talking about changing his drinking habits, or making often unconvincing promises to do so, but is actually doing something about it. These patients are at the 'action' stage in the well-known Prochaska and DiClemente model of changing patterns of addictive behaviour.[73]

Finally, the patient is involving some third party (family member, clinic staff, friend, colleague or probation officer) for the specific purpose of strengthening a resolve that he knows – and they know - is often tenuous, varies from one day to another, and frequently fails altogether.

The last three paragraphs, very slightly shortened, are taken from a review published in 2000.[74] A 2016 paper by Newton-Howes et al (hereinafter referred to as the New Zealand study) correctly noted that although the review hypothesised that the effectiveness of disulfiram relied on these three mutually reinforcing factors, it did not provide any empirical evidence for the hypothesis.[75] The New Zealand study was designed to find out whether such evidence existed and it

---

[73] Peteet JR, Brenner S, Curtiss D, Ferrigno M, Kauffman J. A stage of change approach to addiction in the medical setting. Gen Hosp Psychiat 1998 Sep;20(5):267-73.
[74] Brewer C, Meyers RJ, Johnsen J. Does disulfiram help to prevent relapse in alcohol abuse? CNS Drugs 2000;14:329-341
[75] Newton-Howes G, Levack WM, McBride S, Gilmor M, Tester R. Non-physiological mechanisms influencing disulfiram treatment of alcohol use disorder: A grounded theory study. Drug Alc Depend 2016;165:126-31.

succeeded. Fourteen patients taking supervised disulfiram as part of an outpatient treatment programme were asked about their attitudes to treatment and in particular about the part played in it by disulfiram. Questioned about the deterrent effect, six of the 14 reported that they had not tested out the DAR because they were sufficiently convinced of its reality by hearing about it from clinic staff or other patients. One patient said that he had been persuaded by patients who had experienced the DAR. "Because I think - if it was just as simple as me believing, I'd just start thinking, I wonder if it's a placebo?". Of the eight patients who did risk drinking, all but two experienced a DAR that was sufficiently unpleasant to deter them from further experiments but the subsequent behaviour of those two patients is both interesting and encouraging. Instead of using the inadequate level of ALDH inhibition as a reason to drop out of treatment, or even to criticise the treatment for its ineffectiveness, they accepted dose increases until the DAR was sufficient to deter them. One reported that while taking an inadequate dose, he could drink most of a bottle of vodka before he started feeling ill but stopped drinking once on an adequate dose. This slightly heart-warming story embodies a very simple principle that is taken for granted in most areas of pharmacological treatment: if an effective, evidence-based drug doesn't produce the expected effect, try increasing the dose. Yet several clinicians who use and recommend disulfiram behave as if it were an exception to this very elementary rule.

Another important feature of disulfiram treatment, confirmed by this study, is the way in which disulfiram effectively removes one of the most annoying features of being an alcoholic - the endless internal arguments and conversations that patients have with themselves almost every minute of the day about whether they should or shouldn't drink. Some patients described it as a sort of "internal homunculus that demanded alcohol". Disulfiram replaced those endless ruminations and temptations with a mind-set in which alcohol was "simply no longer an option". One patient described how, when he wasn't taking disulfiram, after all the internal arguments, "at the end of it, I just go 'fuck it, fuck it'… When I'm on Antabuse, it's just like. Well, I can't".

While half the patients admitted that they had tried to manipulate the supervision process in order to drink, they all recognised that taking disulfiram meant – and signified - "choosing to have a day without alcohol". Taking disulfiram not only guaranteed abstinence for the next few days but also made it more likely that they would seriously think about their drinking habits. "Rather than abstinence being a half-hearted commitment – a decision with shifting boundaries – disulfiram made the decision not to drink absolute….".

"Somewhat counter-intuitively, rather than restricting decision-making autonomy, *choosing to take disulfiram was described by many participants as empowering or even liberating. Disulfiram gave back control over life events by removing the weight of continued rumination on drinking and drinking decisions".* (our italics) Another patient stated: "I didn't realise what a positive step it was to empower me, to give me some strength back… something to build on".

The New Zealand study also confirmed the importance of the third of our hypothesised components – the integration of disulfiram with social support and encouragement from community, clinic or family members. "Many expressed concerns about letting others down if they relapsed to drinking...this being a major motivator for maintaining a regular disulfiram regime" They welcomed the combined biopsychosocial approach to their problems, both valuing the counselling and social support and recognising that disulfiram enabled them to remain abstinent for long enough to benefit from them. "This suggests that the social structure in place around delivery of [disulfiram] was key in ensuring its effectiveness in supporting long-term abstinence".

"11 participants in this study reported disulfiram as having contributed significantly to their on-going recovery...all participants recommended it as a treatment option worth trying, and one worth introducing earlier as an option in treatment of alcohol dependency rather than being used as a last resort". It is also therapeutically and philosophically significant that despite the quintessentially medical nature of disulfiram itself, "there was a notable absence of participants having a biomedical explanation" for their alcoholism. "They did not say: I have the disease and therefore need to take a pill as the cure."

In all areas of medicine (especially the 'Complementary and Alternative' variety) placebo effects and non-specific effects are much more prevalent and powerful than many health professionals realise – or are willing to admit. The two types of effect are very different and sometimes non-specific factors have the greater impact. In alcoholism, especially in patients seeking treatment for the first time, the most important non-specific factor is symbolic rather than practical: the act of presenting oneself - and thus in some sense, submitting or surrendering oneself – for treatment.

Studies such as the previously-discussed 'treatment vs advice' comparison demonstrate that supposedly non-therapeutic components of a programme can have large and beneficial effects but other studies show that as in giving up cigarette smoking, many alcoholics give up drinking[76] (or in some cases, become controlled and moderate drinkers[77]) without any treatment at all.[78] This good news is not universally welcomed among addiction professionals. As one researcher notes, spontaneous recovery is "not understood and largely challenged by self-help group members and professionals working in the field of substance abuse. So strong is the supposition of the process of recovering as a life-long condition that requires treatment and/or a self-help group for on-going support and rehabilitation that recovery on one's own is given little credence. Yet there is growing

---

[76] Roizen R, Fillmore KM. Some notes on the new paradigmatic environment of "natural remission" studies in alcohol research. Subst Use Misuse. 2001 Sep;36(11):1443-65.

[77] Dawson DA, Grant BF, Stinson FS, Chou PS, Huang B, Ruan WJ. Recovery from DSM-IV alcohol dependence: United States, 2001-2002. Addiction. 2005 Mar;100(3):281-92.

[78] Sobell LC, Klingemann HK, Toneatto T, Sobell MB, Agrawal S, Leo GI. Alcohol and drug abusers' perceived reasons for self-change in Canada and Switzerland: computer-assisted content analysis. Subst Use Misuse. 2001 Sep;36(11):1467-500.

empirical evidence that natural recovery not only exists, but may be more prominent than is currently recognized".[79]

It is therefore very likely that a numerically significant proportion of patients who present themselves for treatment might have given up or cut down drinking anyway but felt that they needed some professional contact to symbolise, validate, or otherwise reinforce their decision to do so. This is related to a phenomenon known as the 'healthy complier effect' which tells us a lot about both placebos and compliance. While good compliance with effective treatment (i.e. diligently following 'doctor's orders') leads to better outcomes than half-hearted compliance or leaving treatment, compliance itself, *even to placebos*, is a very important predictor of good outcomes. In other words, and particularly where 'easy' patients are concerned, the nature of the treatment complied with may be much less important than whether the level of compliance with treatment is high or low, probably because good compliers tend to be diligent, health-conscious, well-motivated and well-organised people.[80] These personality traits are useful in most areas of life and are likely to facilitate recovery from any illness, condition or misfortune. In contrast, poor compliers are more likely to be disorganised and short on self-discipline, which is not helpful if they are trying to lose old habits and learn

---

[79] Burman S. The challenge of sobriety: natural recovery without treatment and self-help groups. J Subst Abuse. 1997;9:41-61.
[80] Simpson SH, Eurich DT, Majumdar SR, Padwal RS, Tsuyuki RT, Varney J, Johnson JA. A meta-analysis of the association between adherence to drug therapy and mortality. BMJ. 2006 Jul 1;333(7557):15. Epub 2006 Jun 21.

new ones. That is true whether the new habit is getting used to speaking French instead of only English, or getting used to not drinking and to doing something else instead.

In some cultures, many alcoholics choose to make their submission to religious institutions rather than alcoholism services and a priest, rather than a clinician, is the focus of the symbolism and the validation. At their simplest, these medical and religious pilgrimages reflect the fortunate fact – known to any clinician with even a little experience – that patients will often do things for their doctor that they would not do for themselves (another factor supported by the New Zealand study) and the same is true of religious figures, with whom doctors, especially, still have much more in common than many of us like to admit.[81]

Non-specific effects also include things like consultations, physical examinations, reassurance and blood tests. These non-specific procedures – diagnostic or symbolic rather than overtly therapeutic - can make patients feel very much better very quickly but they are features of most therapeutic encounters and are thus not 'specific' to the treatment in question. Non-specific effects may also reflect spontaneous improvement or recovery and the related concept of 'regression to the mean' – the finding that among a hundred people with, say, high blood pressure or low haemoglobin

---

[81] It is true of nurses, psychologists and counsellors as well, though often to a lesser extent. Many modern doctors may be keen to stress that they are only members of a team but many of their patients appear to retain strongly hierarchical attitudes to treatment personnel.

levels, a significant proportion will return to normal within a few months without treatment.

Placebo effects are additional to non-specific effects. They are the effects of the patient's perception of, and faith in, a particular pharmacological, surgical or (in broad terms) psychotherapeutic intervention, regardless of whether or not that intervention has any benefit over and above the effects of an appropriate placebo intervention. Many standard interventions in alcoholism do not confer that additional benefit, or confer it only at very marginal levels. Placebo effects can make clinicians, as well as patients, feel much better. We all like to think that we are able to help our patients because we possess specific knowledge, and that this knowledge is a powerful and specific tool. Our patients like to think that too and the result can be a mutual therapeutic delusion that may not be helpful in the long run. Randomised Controlled Trials are specifically designed to test therapeutic claims, which is why they have not always been welcomed in alcoholism, since many of those claims originate in institutions and clinics that offer only one type of treatment that is not supported by robust evidence.

Powerful placebo effects are most likely to be seen in conditions that have a significant psychological component. Depression is a case in point, especially since it is often part of a 'dual diagnosis' and many alcoholics receive prescriptions for drugs that are supposed to relieve it. Bearing in mind that the more rigorous the controlled trial, the smaller will be the likely difference between placebo and active wings, the difference in effectiveness between antidepressants and suitable placebos in comparative trials is rarely more than about 15% and usually nearer half that. The difference also seems to have become smaller over the last couple of decades.[82] Where an active placebo is used (i.e. a drug that has some mild but obvious side-effects but is not thought to have any therapeutic effect) thus making it more difficult for doctors or patients to guess which group they have been allocated to, the difference is further reduced. What applies to antidepressants also applies, surprisingly, to a common type of back surgery. In an ageing population, many people have back pain apparently related to osteoporosis and the progressive collapse of vertebrae. Vertebroplasty - pumping bone-cement into the crumbling vertebrae in the hope of propping them up and preventing further crumbling - is a relatively simple procedure and to backache-afflicted patients, it sounds like a good idea, though backache is quite often a marker for more general discontents. In fee-per-item health services, it sounds like a good idea to hospitals, surgeons and their accountants as well and it has become quite popular. True to the spirit of science, sceptical enquiry and the null hypothesis, orthopaedic researchers tried to find out how much of the considerable improvement that often follows this procedure is due to placebo and non-specific effects. The answer is that they account for a very large proportion. Patients who only had a small incision under local anaesthetic did as well as those who had the cement as well. "There were significant reductions in overall pain in both study groups at each

---

[82] Cuijpers P, Cristea IA. What if placebo effect explained all the activity of depression treatments? World Psychiat 2015; 14, 310-11.

follow-up assessment [but there was] no beneficial effect of vertebroplasty as compared with a sham procedure in patients with painful osteoporotic vertebral fractures, at 1 week or at 1, 3, or 6 months after treatment".[83] There were similar results in trials of keyhole surgery for arthritis of the knee.[84]

More relevant to addiction treatment are the numerous studies of counselling that show as much as fourfold variations[85] in effectiveness and treatment retention between the best counsellors and the worst.[86] Equally significant is the finding that the differences between counsellors seem to have little to do with the differences in their theoretical orientation. The most important therapeutic component of counselling seems to be the nature of the patient-therapist relationship. Since the quality of this relationship is not something that can be easily tested or demonstrated by professional examinations, or easily and predictably imparted in training, it follows that it is largely a chance feature and thus another non-specific or placebo component of treatment. It may be related to charisma, in a general sense, but

---

[83] Buchbinder R1, Osborne RH, Ebeling PR, Wark JD, Mitchell P, Wriedt C, Graves S, Staples MP, Murphy B. A randomized trial of vertebroplasty for painful osteoporotic vertebral fractures. N Engl J Med. 2009 Aug 6;361(6):557-68.

[84] Moseley JB, O'Malley K, Petersen NJ, et al. A controlled trial of arthroscopic surgery for osteoarthritis of the knee. N Engl J Med. 2002;347:81-8.

[85] Najavitz L, Weiss R. Variations in therapist effectiveness in the treatment of patients with substance use disorders: an empiricial review. Addiction 1994;89:679-688.

[86] Project MATCH Research Group. Therapist Effects in Three Treatments for Alcohol Problems Psychother Res 1998;8,4,

charismatic therapists can, unfortunately, be damaging as well as helpful.

It is now regarded as unethical for doctors to prescribe placebos deliberately without patient awareness or consent[87] and therefore very few doctors realise just how powerful the placebo effect can be. Since everybody in the business of healing likes to think that their particular skills have contributed to a happy outcome, they also tend to be reluctant to recognise just how large a proportion of any improvement may be due to placebo and non-specific factors, or to other matters that are outside their control, or that were never part of the original treatment plan. Here is an instructive case-history with which to end this chapter.

> One of the recurrent alcoholic offenders in the probation-linked disulfiram programme described in Ch. 10 told me that he was staying dry out of prison for the first time in many years. This caused me a little silent self-congratulation, but it soon turned out that factors other than my clinical skills and the ingenious treatment programme were probably also involved. His usual probation officer had left the area and he had been allocated a new one, who therefore had to read his file from the beginning. Before doing so, she made a remark which indicated that she assumed him to be in his mid-40s. Since he was barely 30, this shocked him into a realisation that alcohol was really damaging him in a way that he had not previously considered: his appearance. At his next

---

[87] Which naturally leads to a much-reduced placebo effect but may not necessarily remove it altogether. Some patients responded so well to openly-prescribed placebo tablets that they refused to believe that they really were placebos.

clinic visit, the shock was still very evident. While the programme could take some credit for keeping him sober until he met his new probation officer, it was probably her chance, unplanned and entirely non-specific remark that played a large part in helping him to stay that way for many months, as he did.

Chapter 8. INTERNATIONAL EXPERTS WHO ROUTINELY USE DISULFIRAM.
Proceedings of the Copenhagen Round-Table Disulfiram Symposium of 1996

Participants: Hannu Alho (Finland), Mats Berglund (Sweden), Colin Brewer (Great Britain), Jonathan Chick (Great Britain), H. Enghusen-Poulsen (Denmark), Peter Geerlings (The Netherlands), Finn Hardt (Denmark), Jon Johnsen (Norway), Otto Lesch (Austria), Flavio Poldrugo (Italy), Johan Zierau (Denmark).

[Editorial note. Inevitably, some issues discussed here also appear elsewhere in the book. The discussion has been only slightly edited – e.g. using 'disulfiram' rather than 'Antabuse' throughout – and not all references to published or impending papers could be traced. In a few places where the transcript was confusing, I could not always contact the speaker to clarify it and simply omitted the words or sentence. Finn Hardt, who convened the meeting, died of cancer not long afterwards. He was a gastroenterologist - one of many whose interest in alcoholism arose from their daily contact with its serious medical consequences. He hoped that the proceedings would be published but the journals I approached thought them either unsuitable or too long. Travel expenses were covered by Dumex, the Danish manufacturers of disulfiram but participants did not receive any fees.]

FINN HARDT

This is a good time to look at current issues surrounding the use of disulfiram to the treatment of alcohol problems. It is almost exactly 50 years since the first work was published on the clinical trial done by Martenson-Larsen here in Copenhagen. We now know much more about the metabolism of disulfiram and its toxicity and we know what side effects to look out for. This should help us to discuss guidelines. The main problem, I think, when you are discussing the clinical use of disulfiram, is that there are lots of people who have had both good and bad experiences with it. Swift[88] is the latest of the many reviewers claiming that randomised controlled clinical trials of efficacy showed no improvement, or short-term improvement only and that it can only be used in selected patients. However if you look at the literature on the new anti-craving medicines, you can find similar papers asking; does it have any clinical effects? Who should be treated and for how long?

In order that we do not discuss just one point, I have sent you some of the questions. I think they are not the only questions to be discussed but they will provide a thread through our debate. The first thing to discuss is whether disulfiram really does work. Does it work in short-term therapy (defined as less than three months) or long-term therapy (defined as years)? I think that now we can take some comments. It's a very broad question. We'll start with you Chick

---

[88] Swift RM. Medications and alcohol craving. Alcohol Res Health. 1999;23(3):207-13.

CHICK
Well, there are some randomised controlled studies which have shown its efficacy. However, the studies that have shown effectiveness have supervised the disulfiram in some way. That's my reading of the literature. The longest (there is only one study, I think going beyond one year) would be one of the Azrin studies. Otherwise we've only got studies showing efficacy up to 6 months. It certainly is my practice to suggest six months but often patients request to continue longer. I've been fortunate in not having any experience of some of the rare side-effects which had been reported with long-term use.

HARDT
Would anyone else like to discuss long-term use?

BERGLUND
I would like to mention that we have just presented some of our own studies. They are not randomised studies, but naturalistic designs, in a two-year outpatient treatment programme. At that time, about 90% of Swedish alcoholics got disulfiram. At the present time, it's about 50%. In the naturalistic design with a four-year follow-up after disulfiram treatment in those using disulfiram for more than one year, there was a successful outcome in 75% of the cases. In those using it for less than 12 months, the success rate was 31%. However, this is an old study and on this issue of long-term treatment, it's very difficult to do randomised controlled trials.

LESCH

There was another study, published in 1985 in a German book. We too did a prospective naturalistic study in 45 areas of Austria, looking at all patients who were admitted to any hospital psychiatric ward and diagnosed as alcohol dependent. Then we visited these people at home and have studied them for 18 years. The last report from 1994/1995 is not yet published but the patients that were admitted were alcohol dependent and patients who had disulfiram responded better than those who didn't. If a patient has severe somatic withdrawal symptoms, they are admitted to hospital. In most cases, the patients had a good social background, no severe personality disorder and agreed to the aim of sobriety. We put them on disulfiram for a month and it worked.

BREWER

There is always a problem with patients who don't take disulfiram because you would expect patients who decline disulfiram to have a worse prognosis than those who accept it. To some extent, the people who agree to take disulfiram willingly are, on the whole, relatively easy patients. Part of the skill in treatment is to persuade people who are not very keen on disulfiram to accept it in the first place. Unless you do some sort of randomised study, it is difficult to be sure that differences in outcome don't simply reflect differences in the patients. However, I think there are two reasons why we should consider it for long term as well as short-term treatment.

Firstly, if patients with other conditions keep relapsing unless they are on a particular treatment, then we continue to prescribe that treatment, whether it is antidepressants, lithium or anything else and I don't see that disulfiram is any different. From time to time you may stop the treatments to see whether they still need it and if patients keep relapsing, they need a further course. Secondly, we can draw some comfort from a trial done in a rather different context. Chan[89] studied the effect of naltrexone in heroin addicts who had to take it as a condition of probation. These were reluctant patients, but they took it for a year because if they didn't take it for a year, they went back to prison. The compliance rate was very high and the success rate was very high: 75% were still opiate-free a year later, compared with 25% in the otherwise identical programme that didn't include naltrexone. Even more interesting is that after two years, a year after they had stopped the naltrexone, some of them had clearly got into the habit of abstinence, because most of them didn't relapse straight away. I think that if you can persuade people to take disulfiram for long enough and even without a lot of psychological treatment, some of them will just get used to abstinence, perhaps for the first time in their lives and they don't need to take it afterwards. So I think there is a case for long-term treatment as well.[90]

JOHNSEN
In Norway, female therapists commented that most of the studies have been done in men. They say that they have not

---

[89] Chan KY. The Singapore naltrexone community-based project for heroin addicts compared with drugfree community-based program: the first cohort. J Clin Med 1996;3:87-92

[90] This hypothesis is supported by the results of the long-term OLITA studies.

had as much experience in giving it to women, and wonder if it could have a different adverse effect profile to that in men. The Addiction Society also discussed whether you can prescribe disulfiram to young patients. I am thinking about the age group between 20 and 25 years. It's very important to get control over their drinking because they need to continue education, to settle in society and so on. There needs to be some debate about the use of disulfiram in young people and in women.

POLDRUGO

At first, in Italy, we had only a standard programme of detoxification until 1979. Then we introduced a programme that included disulfiram treatment for most of the patients. About 50% took it and we had a great decrease in mortality after we started using disulfiram.

HARDT

Any more comments at this point?

ZIERAU

How do we define long-term treatment? If over a period of three years a patient has ten relapses, and you use disulfiram in between, is that long-term or short-term treatment? Of course, we say in our clinics that we only offer disulfiram to people who want to stay sober, but not all people want to stay without alcohol for the same length of time. Many people who have had relapses say they will never drink again. So is it meaningful to talk about long-term or short-term treatment? Many of the patients themselves choose long-term abstinence without necessarily having long-term treatment.

LESCH

I agree. We did one trial with 56 sober alcohol dependent outpatients. They took disulfiram regularly for two years and during visits we analysed their breath and measured blood pressure. We were considering the possible side-effects of disulfiram and included the discussion of sexual function as one of the topics. We designed a trial where two researchers went to the homes of the patients and did separate interviews. The interviews included questions about partnership, sexual behaviour and other social aspects. They lasted for 3 to 4 hours and during the interviews, patients were also asked questions about their drinking behaviour.

Of the 56 patients, only 20% said they drank no alcohol. Of the others, 18 said they drank two times a year. 10 said 1 to 2 times per month; and eight reported drinking on more occasions. When they came to the outpatient unit, they were all sober. The study highlighted two different patterns of disulfiram intake and drinking behaviour. The first group of patients felt it better to take disulfiram to control rather than prevent drinking. When they got a reaction they would stop. Then they would start again, and so on. The second group would stop taking disulfiram totally for 10 days, leave the village and drink very heavily for two days, then they would go back to the village, resume disulfiram and return to our unit.

JOHNSEN

In a study that I was involved with several years ago, cognitive behavioural therapy was the main treatment. We compared a minimal intervention group with a group that received three months of group therapy. At the end of the study after two years, we looked at all the patients who had used disulfiram. Some had used it for more than three months, but very many patients had used it flexibly, in high-risk situations,[91] for example during summer holidays. The patients who used disulfiram did better than the patients who didn't use it. It was quite interesting to see that whether or not they received cognitive behavioural therapy, they managed this flexible use of disulfiram very well.

POLDRUGO

I also use disulfiram in a flexible treatment programme. Patients may stop taking it for a few days, maybe drinking with a family member. What is important with disulfiram is how closely the patient can be monitored. For example, you may not need a marker for alcohol as you will know very soon if they are drinking again, because a member of the family will tell you. Otherwise, in my experience, even a good clinician may not easily recognise if someone has been drinking. It can take some time before you get major signs. With disulfiram you find out quickly if they have been drinking. At the very least the family member will call you and report that the patient has stopped disulfiram. General practitioners may treat alcoholics themselves or refer them to a specialist unit. The patient who is not seriously impaired may decide not to go to the specialist unit but can still be treated using a programme at the clinic in conjunction with his GP. This means that the GP can play his proper role. This is a helpful partnership because it allows the doctor to work

---

[91] cf. Öjehagen and Berglund. Op cit.

from his practice, while maintaining a good relationship with the programme.

BERGLUND

We have done follow-up studies of these outpatients. When a treatment programme ends, then disulfiram consumption decreases very considerably. We stopped all our patients' treatment after two years, but it was possible for them to go to other physicians or clinics after that. During the following two years, only 50% of the subjects used disulfiram at any time. When we finish a ten-year follow-up study, it will probably show that it is quite unusual to use disulfiram for long periods. I think it's really during an intensive treatment phase, which could last for two years or more, that patients really use disulfiram regularly.[92] I know of other studies, including those mentioned by Poldrugo that also described this flexible use of disulfiram, even if abstinence was the goal. As a matter of fact, in our studies, those who changed between abstinence and controlled drinking used disulfiram better than the abstinence-only group. I think with this approach that you mentioned earlier with family involvement, we could reproduce the same data in our study.

BREWER

I published a couple of individual case reports of patients using disulfiram, in one case for about 10 years and in another case about 15 years. The 15-year one was very interesting. He still takes disulfiram under his wife's supervision on Mondays and Tuesdays and maybe Wednesdays, because his drinking problem occurred only

---

[92] Again, in keeping with the OLITA results.

during the week. He never had a problem at the weekend. The disulfiram wears off by Friday. He and his wife enjoy a bottle of wine on Saturday and Sunday and he takes it again on Monday. He has been doing this for 15 years and is very well on it. Regarding compliance, I think that because disulfiram is such an effective drug – because it really does work for most patients – an important part of the family education and feedback is to tell them not only about supervising the disulfiram but also about the little tricks that patients sometimes use to evade it, such as swapping the tablets for something else, and about the importance of dissolving the tablets. Azrin is one of the few researchers who really stressed the importance of dissolving disulfiram and seeing people actually swallow it. It's so easy for patients to pretend to swallow it and that's a common cause of relapse.

LESCH
I'd like to stress the role of the GP. Only four or five percent of alcohol dependent patients go to see other professionals. Most of them are treated by the GP and will never see a specialist. What we need is a manual for the use of allied health professionals as well as GPs. We need this not only to avoid mistakes but because health professionals are worried about possible misuse of disulfiram. For example that a wife may surreptitiously put it in her husband's coffee. We need a real manual discussing what kind of patient, in what kind of situation and for how long a GP can prescribe disulfiram. There are lots of people, living in little villages, who want to get sober for two, three or four weeks. They want to stop drinking but still sit with their friends in the restaurant and

other social situations. Disulfiram helps them. They are willing to take it and the GP can manage these patients because they need no intensive psychotherapeutic help, though they may need simple counselling.

GEERLINGS

I agree with Dr Lesch. We found in Amsterdam that only 5% of alcoholic patients come to the specialist or ambulatory clinics and 1% to inpatients. About 50% visit the GP. The GP often doesn't discuss the problem when he starts treatment. In maybe 10% of the cases, he prescribes disulfiram without any supervision. There is enough evidence to show that disulfiram is most effective when its consumption is supervised. We have to provide manuals, guidelines or a training programme to ensure that disulfiram will be used effectively.

ALHO

Disulfiram could be used more effectively by GPs. It is rarely used in Finland, much less than in Denmark and other countries, and usually only by specialists. This could be because GPs do not know how to use disulfiram correctly. When the patient visits the GP and is prescribed disulfiram, the GP usually just gives out the prescription and says: 'Take these pills and then you cannot drink'. Some kind of protocol or set of guidelines would be very useful. It should highlight some of the points addressed already today as well as using it in women and young people and the possible side-effects following long-term use. I think that these are the main issues for GPs.

CHICK

I have letters from general practitioners which say things like: 'This patient has come to ask for disulfiram. Please would you see him or her'. Another letter may say: 'This patient has an alcohol problem. Please advise if disulfiram is suitable'. We have a three-month waiting list, so I write or telephone the GP and then I send instructions through the post. These instructions explain how to set up a supervision system. Sometimes it works and sometimes we see the patients three months later anyway. In the British health service, there is an increasing use of the nurse based in the general practice. Sometimes the doctor works out some system, perhaps with the employer or the wife, so that the patient visits the nurse three times a week at their general practice site.

HARDT

Shall we discuss the system of control and supervision? Some of you have said that it is essential. Maybe we should discuss the system? Some of us agree that a doctor or nurse should supervise. Others think that anyone is suitable as long as they can do the job. I would like to have some comments on this.

JOHNSEN

I think we have talked about the studies of Azrin and how important it is to involve the family.[93] You have to train and

---

[93] Azrin N, Sissons R, Meyer SR, Godley M. Alcoholism treatment by disulfiram and community reinforcement therapy. J Behav Ther Exper Psychiat 1982;13, 105-112.

teach them, so maybe you have to provide some training material.

BERGLUND

In Sweden, it is generally not regarded as correct to work together with the spouse of the alcoholic in order to increase compliance. I think that this is not a modern approach and it is possible to use disulfiram liaising with different people in different ways. Tim O'Farrell's approach to using disulfiram[94] is a good example but many people and many doctors in Sweden still think that you have to go to a specialist clinic or to the district nurse in order to get disulfiram.

BREWER

We have a little leaflet that explains about family involvement. It explains why supervision is necessary, describes the various tricks that people use and so on. I think that any system that works is useful. Sometimes a combination of the family and the doctor will succeed where the family alone fails. George Bernard Shaw joked that faith in God hasn't died out in Britain, it has simply been transferred to doctors. A lot of patients will do things for doctors that they will not do for their wives or husbands. So I usually say to my supervisors: 'If he refuses disulfiram, please telephone me'. I then call the patient and ask him what he thinks he is doing. They don't always resume disulfiram but it's quite helpful and people will often accept it just

---

[94] O'Farrell TJ, Bayog RD. Antabuse contracts for married alcoholics and their spouses: a method to maintain antabuse ingestion and decrease conflict about drinking. J Subst Abuse Treat. 1986;3(1):1-8.

because you're a doctor. It seems to me silly not to use that kind of magic if we all have it.

JOHNSEN

I have also read and heard several American therapists, for instance Galanter, who use disulfiram in conjunction with family therapy, and have succeeded. As has been mentioned, it is difficult to do randomised trials but clinical experience is that it is an effective approach. There are also studies by a Canadian group using calcium carbimide [cyanamide].[95] They are very interested in attribution theory and keen that patients should not attribute all their achievements to the tablets alone.

LESCH

The quality and style of treatment varies in different countries. As you know, there are some countries who are strongly influenced by Alcoholics Anonymous (AA) and which have no additional treatment programs. However, they may have education programs, and with these education programs it is possible to give medication, like disulfiram. There are also countries where there is extensive psychotherapeutic support. In our country, we have regular meetings with the GPs. Not only supervision of disulfiram is discussed but also psychotherapy. In small towns, sometimes people have to go to AA because there is no other alternative. They may have five days of in-patient treatment and then

---

[95] Annis HM, Peachey JE. The use of calcium carbimide in relapse prevention counselling: results of a randomized controlled trial. Br J Addict. 1992 Jan;87(1):63-72.

nothing. In this field, I think it's very difficult to define a level of supervision because of the differences between regions. Each case must be considered individually.

BERGLUND
I think the expectations of patients about treatment of their addiction are very important. In Sweden about 10 to 15 years ago, patients usually expected that they should start on disulfiram as the treatment of choice. Then attitudes changed and if you had a problem with alcohol, then you would join AA or go into Minnesota-model treatment. There are obviously very different approaches today. Disulfiram is not now the most common approach. Ten years ago, the nurse just put the patient on disulfiram without discussing it with the doctor. At present, it's unusual for them to make disulfiram the first choice. Now it's changing again, away from the Minnesota model to perhaps using anti-craving agents. Incidentally, 10 years ago in Sweden, it was not necessary to be a doctor in order to prescribe disulfiram. A social worker could do it without discussing it with any doctor.

POLDRUGO
In my experience we have two populations of alcoholics. Those who go to the clinic are what I call clinical alcoholics. These people are very impaired. The mortality rate after five years is 30%, so there isn't really an option whether to treat not. You have to make them abstain from alcohol, otherwise you lose them. For these people, we introduced disulfiram at the beginning as the first mode of treatment. In other cases you can bargain. Maybe in some cases you can use

disulfiram and in other cases not. The treatment of alcoholics is usually a long-term, dynamic process. I suggest that disulfiram is used in a sustained, supported programme. You cannot simply tell alcoholics not to drink if they have many additional problems. You need to create a network of support and give disulfiram in conjunction with the support.

CHICK
This probably doesn't only apply to the taking of the disulfiram. When you are struggling between something that you still quite enjoy and the alternative, which is giving it up, there has got to be a reward or some other pressure. We feel that we should maximise and clarify the pressures and rewards of patients. This is where disulfiram supervision comes in. Of course, it's fairly obvious if there is coercion. If there is some immediate threat, then the person making the threat, as long as the relationship with them is not too bad, is a good person to supervise the disulfiram. This may include pressure from the place of work or from a wife.

There is only a small proportion, perhaps half of our disulfiram patients, who also have such a distinct motivation. Elsewhere we take advantage of them not wanting to let down the group at the clinic. Seeing the nurse, and being given a little encouragement three times a week, gives the supervision some added value. Treatment has to have that added value for the patient. If there is no system like that, we usually say to a patient that we are not sure whether simply taking disulfiram at home is going to work. That's our experience. There are those who are very exceptional and organised and we will let them take it without supervision.

Otherwise we tend to say: don't bother with disulfiram. In our experience, just giving you disulfiram to take home, when your motivations are so fluctuating, means that you will probably use it for two weeks and then stop it. Why not start on some other scheme?

LESCH
We define these patients as Type I patients [in the Lesch typology] and say: 'OK, you have to go to a self-help group, to AA perhaps, or a similar group but you can also get disulfiram'. This group may also get acamprosate as well and then they get no psychotherapeutic approach but only counselling and supervision, nothing else. There is another group of patients who only need psychotherapeutic approaches. These may involve psychotherapy in addition to family therapy. We never give disulfiram in these cases. For us it is very clear who will get what kind of support, what kind of therapy, and who will not get it. 7% of alcohol dependent patients respond very well with a combination of AA and disulfiram. This combination may double the sobriety rate in these patients.

HARDT
What do you do when you start your family therapy without disulfiram? Can you keep them sober initially?

LESCH
It's like the concept of naltrexone. The concept of naltrexone is damage limitation. The concept of family therapy is to introduce interactions between family members. Family

therapy should be an interactive process and disulfiram administration may disturb some families.

GEERLINGS

About your question of how to increase compliance. I think that this is not an issue only for psychiatrists. It is for the whole medical profession. There are a lot of studies and publications on the subject. There are books on evidence-based medicine which discuss how to make telephone contact and things like counselling that can improve compliance. I think it is not really specific to psychiatry or alcohol treatment. What matters is how we can improve compliance in specific cases.

HARDT

We have various forms of disulfiram but I think we should discuss the question of how much we should give. The dose should be sufficiently effective that if someone drinks when taking it, then they get a reaction. In Denmark we usually increase the dose if they drink on disulfiram, so some patients may get quite a high dose.

JOHNSEN

In many review articles, they conclude that the results were negative when using disulfiram. The articles often refer to the study of Fuller et al[96] with 500 male patients. I'm not quite sure if the dosage in that study was high enough to induce disulfiram reactions to alcohol. They used ordinary tablets

---

[96] Fuller. *Op Cit*

which have poor bioavailability compared to more soluble formulations.

ALHO

Do you know of any studies, or do you have experience that if disulfiram is given on a controlled basis and in dissolved form, so that we know for sure that the patient has taken the medicine, the patients actually get the recommended dose?

BREWER

It's quite clear that some patients can take large doses of disulfiram without any reaction to alcohol. There are very few publications on this topic. Lenz[97] wrote a paper showing that some patients with liver disease may not convert disulfiram to its presumed active metabolite and the same point is made by Johansson.[98] However, I have seen patients without any liver disease and who I am quite sure were getting disulfiram, sometimes as in-patients. In other cases, I have checked as much as I can with the family. I agree with Finn Hardt that the thing to do in such cases is to increase the dose, but you can increase it up to 600 or 800 mg a day and still not get any response. On the other hand, this is true of almost all drugs. For most people a small dose of disulfiram is adequate because if they are taking it regularly, they don't usually take the risk of drinking. That's why disulfiram

---

[97] Lenz VH. Zur ursache der fehlenden Antabus-alcohol reaction. Wien Clin Wochenschr 1957, Sept 27

[98] Johansson B. A review of the pharmacokinetics and pharmacodynamics of disulfiram and its metabolites. Acta Psychiatr Scand Suppl. 1992;369:15-26.

implants work very well for some people. It's not because of the blood levels of disulfiram, which are undetectable.

BERGLUND

I do agree with you that some people may need to have larger doses of disulfiram but the reason why people can still drink when taking disulfiram could be, for example, that there is an interaction with other drugs that the patient is taking. We don't know much about drug interactions of disulfiram. Maybe they try to avoid taking the drug and we don't know about it. I think you could start with 400 mg a day for a week and then either give 200 mg or 400 mg three times a week. I don't increase the doses – not for pharmacological reasons but for psychological or psychosocial ones.

CHICK

When the family say: 'He's been drinking and he didn't have a reaction', the first question is, was he really taking the tablets? Often the wife will say: 'Oh yes yes. I see him take it every day'. Then you ask the question: 'Well in the last three days, did you actually see him take the correct tablet?' Then she goes and discovers that there are some aspirin tablets that he has taken instead. So you have a meeting with the family and you say: 'Well, where do we go from here?' And you ask the patient: 'In principle, do you really want to have disulfiram treatment? Okay, you do? Well, let's get a better system so that you actually take it'. If he has been taking it (and I agree with Brewer that some people on 200 mg daily don't get much reaction) then you say: 'Do you still want to continue with this treatment? If you do, then we need to increase the dose, don't we?' There are nevertheless a few people who, even when you go up to 400 mg daily still don't get any reaction, so we usually leave it after that.

LESCH
There are some patients who actually like to drink with disulfiram because they like to get high acetaldehyde levels. They take high doses of disulfiram and drink a lot of alcohol and they don't like it if we stop the medication. So if the patient is drinking and taking disulfiram, we discontinue disulfiram.[99]

JOHNSEN
We know that disulfiram is metabolised to an active metabolite that inhibits the various ALDH enzymes. When formed, this would create an alcohol reaction and from other studies it has been shown that where there is severe liver disease, some of the enzymes which are involved in the metabolism are too weak to produce these active metabolites. This may mean that there could be lower expression of the alcohol reaction in those patients. Also in healthy people, if for some reason the level of the enzymes is low, that may be the reason for the absence of the alcohol reaction.

POLDRUGO
I want to make a comment about how we give disulfiram in our programmes. We give it during the weekly sessions of group therapy, so we have the health professional dealing

---

[99] I have come across only a single patient who persistently drank on disulfiram but he only took about half a unit, just before going to bed, because he liked the sensation of slight warmth and thought it helped him to sleep. Otherwise, he abstained.

with the case monitoring who is and who is not taking disulfiram. The decision to take the drug is made between a number of people including a health professional, family member and a member of the group. We may decide not to give it because there is some real medical risk but otherwise, we continue and we can discuss with the patients whether to increase the dose. This is always a bargaining process. I think it's really the way that you give it that makes the difference. For us, one key factor in our programme is that we were also able to get involved in the treatment of patients who had no network support, for example, no family. So the group can act as a substitute or reinforcement for the family and can thus produce positive results using this drug.

JOHNSEN
I would also like to say something about the possibility of monitoring compliance with treatment. One way is to analyse, using pharmacokinetics, the production of the active metabolites. Another way is to follow the inactivation of one of the enzymes involved in the metabolism of ethanol. This can be done using white or red blood cells. For instance some researchers have found a good correlation between enzyme inhibition in the liver and the enzyme inhibition in white blood cells. This is currently an expensive way of monitoring treatment but it would be a way to ensure that the drug hits the target.[100]

---

[100] The Zenalyser (Fletcher K. Disulfiram and the Zenalyser®: teaching an old dog new tricks. Alcohol Alcohol. 2015; 50(2):255-6) may make this much easier.

GEERLINGS.
Can we agree with what Berglund told us? We normally begin treatment with 400 mg a day (of course there are exceptions) then maybe one week or two weeks later we can use 200 mg daily. I use this schedule but what do other people do?

POLDRUGO
We are also using 400 mg a day to start. One problem of the programme is if they are not continuously supervised. The doctor tends to decrease the dose, not because the original dose is unnecessary but because of pressure from the patient not to take it. So the doctors give half or a quarter of the first dose, decreasing to a minimal level but this is a supervision issue. About the reaction to disulfiram, I know that some people can drink while taking it. I do not know for how long they can do it. In my experience, I haven't really treated people who drink and take disulfiram for a long period. Maybe two weeks but not longer.

For a time, we used to observe the disulfiram-alcohol reaction in the clinic. This was very useful for two reasons. First of all, you see the reaction immediately, if it occurs, so you know the disulfiram dose is adequate. Secondly, you can monitor some of the effects. We found in some patients there was no immediate effect, but the reaction occurred much later. For example, we had two cases of hypotension that occurred four hours after drug administration. We were aware of this and so could monitor it. Sometimes people are not aware of the later effects and that could be very dangerous. Continuous observation is impractical because it takes a lot of time and the doctor must be present.

CHICK

You have reminded me of an important point. I think the information available does not emphasise that there are some delayed aspects to this reaction. One of the deaths that was reported in the 1950s occurred about eight hours after the patient's close observations were completed. It was a patient who had a history of heart disease. With regard to dose, for some reason the British datasheet advises 800 mg on day one, 600 mg on day two and so on to 200 mg daily.[101] I'm not quite sure how this schedule emerged. We give four 200mg tablets on the first day. It's very unusual to get complaints of unwanted effects on the first day, even after such a dose. The unwanted effects, such as drowsiness, and not usually reported until the second week, so maybe it's due to some metabolite.

ENGHUSEN-POULSEN

The experience we have is from looking into the registers of adverse reactions. It is interesting to note that of all the reports compiled by the WHO Collaborating Centre in Sweden, there were 124 reporting a total of 154 adverse drug reactions (spontaneous reports). This was over a period from 1968 to 1991. That's quite a long time, so not many adverse reactions reported every year. It's clearly an underreported

---

[101] The current (2017) UK datasheet recommends starting at 200mg daily, increasing if necessary up to 500mg daily. It also says that alcohol challenges should not be done 'routinely', which seems to imply that they may be done if necessary in particular cases.

subject. However, we were able to extract some data and some patterns from this. Particularly if you look at the figures and tables in the Acta Psychiatrica Supplement,[102] it is quite evident that there is a temporal difference in reporting. You can see there is an early onset of skin reactions along with a peak of liver effects at about 60 days. That declines with time and with long-term treatment. Once the patient has passed this peak period, these effects don't appear again. The neurological reactions, which usually mean peripheral neuropathy, tend to increase with length of treatment. If signs of liver toxicity have not occurred after two or three months they are not likely to occur. Skin reactions will occur very early if they occur at all. Neurological problems tend to increase with increasing time of treatment.

I don't think that disulfiram presents any pattern in adverse reactions that would require intensive surveillance. As with any other drug, one should be observant and note any reactions, be aware of possible side effects, especially liver toxicity and stop the treatment as quickly as possible. This also applies to the neurological problems that can occur with long-term treatment. There are no reports after more than 360 days of treatment, which probably indicates that continuous treatment from more than one year is quite rare. So, in conclusion, I would say that you have to know what the adverse reactions are so that you can monitor them. As well as monitoring patients, you should tell them that if they get skin reactions they should come to the clinic. You should be particularly observant about two months into treatment. Later

---

[102] Acta Psychiatr Scand Suppl. 1992;369

on, in long-term treatment, you should question or maybe examine patients with peripheral neuropathy in mind.

HARDT
Do you recommend any blood tests before starting treatment?

ENGHUSEN-POULSEN
I think there are no tests to predict which patients will react adversely. It is a random process.

GEERLINGS
Do you have any data about women and also pregnancy?

ENGHUSEN-POULSEN
There are no reports on that in the databases. I have no experience myself with pregnant women and treatment for alcoholism. Pregnant women who drink a lot are presumably a high-risk group. I didn't think that disulfiram would have an important role in that context. Such patients require much more intensive treatment with a variety of methods other than drug therapy.

LESCH
I agree, because there are many issues associated with pregnancy. We know nothing about the effects of disulfiram on the baby. I will not give disulfiram during pregnancy.

GEERLINGS
There are publications that say disulfiram can harm the foetus. What do you think?

ENGHUSEN-POULSEN
I think that it will be very difficult to distinguish between the toxic effects of alcohol, of disulfiram or the combination of both drugs in this situation. I would say that the aim of the therapy would be to stop treatment with disulfiram but also to stop drinking. You have a very limited time to achieve this. The problem doesn't exist after the pregnancy.

ZIERAU
If everything else fails and you think that the patient will drink if you don't give disulfiram, what would you recommend?

ENGHUSEN-POULSEN
I would probably give up, to be honest! If possible, I would advise in-patient treatment and closely supervise them. First of all, to see if just achieving abstinence for some time would relieve the problem. Or perhaps to start another sort of therapy. I think that this is a very difficult group to handle. Coming back to your question, I would say: it depends. Late in the pregnancy, I would probably not be so reluctant to give disulfiram as I would be early in the pregnancy. This is not based on any data but simply taking into account organogenesis, which occurs early on. After three or four months, I would not be so concerned with the teratogenic effects. You have to consider the toxic effect of alcohol versus the potential toxic effects of the disulfiram and I think that's an individual judgement that must be made.

ZIERAU

I think that in Denmark, a doctor would give the patient disulfiram in pregnancy if he really had his back against the wall. We have discussed in Denmark whether we could treat these women compulsorily but in that case, I think there is really no way out unless you put them in jail or in a closed psychiatric ward.

ENGHUSEN-POULSEN

This raises another issue. I don't think you can force treatment on these people, at least not in Denmark. In order to do that, they would have to fulfil the legal criteria for compulsory treatment with medication; firstly, they would have to be declared insane. This is mandatory. They would also have to be a danger either to themselves or to other people. Perhaps danger could be invoked if they are pregnant (because of the foetus) but you certainly would have to assure yourself that they really are insane as well, otherwise you cannot force treatment on them

ALHO

I would like to know if you think there is any relationship between dose and occurrence of adverse reactions. As you say, the skin reactions mainly come during the first week. If the recommended starting dose, 800 mg, then 600 mg, 400 mg and 200 mg a day for the first week is followed, might this be a reason for the skin reaction? We start with 400 mg twice a week and we see very few skin reactions.

ENGHUSEN-POULSEN

We don't know the mechanism[103] and we don't know the relation to the daily dose of the initial dose. There are no data available. If you talk about cumulative dose, I would say there is no relationship between the psychiatric side-effects, the cutaneous side-effects or the hepatotoxicity. The steady increase in the neurological symptoms tends to indicate that the cumulative dose is important. Whether it's a true phenomenon or not, we cannot really say for this dose, but that is my interpretation of the curves.

BREWER

It's important to distinguish between at least two types of skin reaction. There may be a proper disulfiram rash. I'm not sure that I've ever seen one. What I have seen is the activation of nickel dermatitis and the treatment of this is not to stop the disulfiram. You carry on with the disulfiram and the rash disappears, because it chelates the nickel and takes it out of circulation. The only such case I have seen happened about two weeks after I had read a paper on it, so I decided to test the theory out and the rash settled down very quickly.

Perhaps this is the time to mention some thoughts about disulfiram hepatotoxicity and nickel? Finn Hardt and I are publishing a paper[104] about disulfiram hepatitis and starting disulfiram in patients with liver disease. Our feeling is that

---

[103] See: Kaaber K, Menne T, Veien N, Baadsgaard O. Some adverse effects of fisulfiram in the treatment of nickel-allergic patients. Dermatosen Beruf Umwelt 1987;38;209-11

[104] Brewer C. Hardt F. Preventing disulfiram hepatitis in alcohol abusers: inappropriate guidelines and the significance of nickel allergy. Addiction Biol 1999;4:303-308

most cases of so-called disulfiram hepatitis are actually due to nickel. The majority of cases reported were in women and yet only a minority of patients taking disulfiram – and probably quite a small minority – are women. Of course, more women get nickel sensitisation because even in these egalitarian days, they wear more costume jewellery. Nickel is very toxic and 10% of people treated for nickel sensitivity with disulfiram get hepatitis. They never die from it because physicians usually examine their patients and notice when they get jaundice. Psychiatrists usually don't and so the patients died because nobody noticed that they turned yellow. No patient has ever died if disulfiram was stopped as soon as jaundice occurred. I think it supports what you were saying – that you can't predict who is going to get an adverse reaction. The only thing you can do is to warn patients that if they get a nasty rash, or their urine turns a strange colour or their toes go numb, they should seek advice straight away. This seems to be the rule with all drugs that occasionally cause serious side effects. It's not something that you can predict. You just tell the patients and the family to let you know if anything goes wrong.

ENGHUSEN-POULSEN
I would like to draw your attention to the safety evaluations we have tried to make. We came up with a rough estimate of adverse drug reactions from disulfiram between 1:200 and 1:2000 per treatment year. That of course gives an underestimate as there is no real definition of what is a treatment reaction but it's neither very frequent nor very infrequent. If we look at mortality, there are 14 deaths reported, which would be approximately one death per 25,000 patients treated

for one year. This is not a high figure. Even if the true figure is 10 times greater, that doesn't really indicate a large problem. So you are facing an intermediate incidence of adverse reactions that is very similar to many other drugs. The relative risk with this treatment is not high. If you know what the adverse reactions are and you know when they occur and you tell the patients about them, I don't foresee any problems. The worst problem of neurological effects occurs with long-term treatment, which may be irreversible.

BREWER
I have seen a few cases of disulfiram neuropathy and with one exception they were all completely reversible. The only exception was one who wasn't diagnosed promptly and wasn't actually under my care at the time. There is one case, published in French, of someone who was on disulfiram for three years and the daily dose was suddenly increased from no particular reason, from 500 mg to 1000mg. Perhaps someone made a clerical error. At that point the patient developed a neuropathy, but it was reversible.

ENGHUSEN-POULSEN
In Denmark, we rarely see treatment periods of more than about a year so I don't think that presents a problem. My point was that if you really go into intense programs for many years, you might see these problems.

JOHNSEN
In Norway, and perhaps all of Europe, there is an increasing problem in that bipolar patients and schizophrenics can also have severe alcohol problems. In Norway we found out that

we can use disulfiram in such cases. Disulfiram can increase dopamine levels in the brain and induce periods of psychosis. I don't think that this is very well documented. There are also warnings about using disulfiram together with atypical new antipsychotic drugs. Often I see serious reactions in patients I'm treating who are using huge amounts of alcohol together with clozapine and other drugs. But I think many of the schizophrenic and bipolar patients need treatment for their alcohol problems, so some of them will gain much benefit from disulfiram.

ENGHUSEN-POULSEN
I have no systematic experience to give you. There are no solid data on the biochemical mechanisms.

BERGLUND
I think this is a very important issue. Larson at al [105] concluded that most of the early reports concern very high doses of disulfiram. We investigated all the cases in our department and we had only one case of psychotic reaction which could be related to disulfiram during 25 years, during which we treated about 3000 patients. So in Sweden, we removed all warnings against using disulfiram in psychotic patients. We maintain that it can be very helpful to use disulfiram in psychotic states.

---

[105] Larson E *et al.* Disulfiram treatment of patients with both alcohol dependence and other psychiatric disorders: A review. Alc Clin Exp Res 1992;16:125-130.

JOHNSEN

Can I just give a comment on nickel sensitivity. It is known that disulfiram is metabolised to carbonyl sulphide and carbonyl sulphide forms a very stable complex with nickel. This complex is very hydrophobic which means that it is readily transported into the central nervous system. This complex with nickel is also carcinogenic. Formation of this compound depends on the metabolism of the individual but I think this is an important point to make.

POLDRUGO

I want to comment on toxicity. We had two cases of toxicity, one acute and one chronic. One involved psychosis in a patient who had taken a large amount of the drug. He needed, I think, two or three months of antipsychotic treatment. The second case, which has been published[106] was of a young person who took a large dose of disulfiram and went into a coma for six months. For the following six months, he had a generalised neuropathy but then recovered. We suspected he was also probably taking cocaine at the time. These are the only two cases I know.

GEERLINGS

I would like to know what the group think about this, because in the "information to the patient" disulfiram is contraindicated in psychosis. If we agree that it is really not contraindicated, I think this is important.

---

[106] I could not contact Prof Poldrugo about the citation but there are a few overdose cases in the literature involving basal ganglia lesions and lengthy but reversible coma, including: Lemoyne S, Raemaekers J, Daems J, Heytens L. Delayed and prolonged coma after acute disulfiram overdose. Acta Neurol Belg. 2009 Sep;109(3):231-4.

CHICK
There is a paper from Kosten and his group in North America, looking at disulfiram and cocaine. This showed a six-fold increase in the availability of the cocaine itself or its active metabolites, though I'm not sure of the implications. Can I just ask about this nickel reaction that has been mentioned? Do some people, because they have worn nickel jewellery for many years, absorb it through the skin or do we take nickel in the diet?

JOHNSEN
Both ways, I think. We have some nickel intake on a daily basis and you also can accumulate it by absorption from skin.

CHICK
Well, we see people with all kinds of nickel perforations on their body. Are they at more risk of this skin reaction or even of liver reaction?

HARDT
We know from women having their ears pierced that about 10% of Danish women are allergic to nickel.

BREWER
I would just like to amplify Geerlings' point about whether we should actually recommend a change in the current advice about disulfiram in cases of psychosis. I have one chronic schizophrenic patient who has periodic excessive drinking, which makes his management difficult. Disulfiram has a beneficial effect on his psychosis only because when he stops drinking, things improve. I think the advice should be no

more than a caution. Perhaps the same applies to pregnancy. We need to justify its use very carefully but I don't think it should be an absolute as opposed to a relative contraindication. I'm not sure if there *are* any absolute contraindications to disulfiram, except known hypersensitivity.

CHICK
I'm surprised to hear that you have taken psychosis out of the Swedish data sheet. I tried to remove it when I was asked by the Journal of Drug Safety to make an update on safety matters. There hasn't been very much published since the excellent report of Larsson et al but there are still some cases being reported. There was one case of catatonia, where the patient was re-exposed to disulfiram and again developed severe catatonia. We found that there were many more psychiatric cases in the WHO databank for some reason, compared to the Danish databank and two of the other reports since 1992 have both been from one unit in India, where they use a lot of disulfiram. Although many patients smoke cannabis in India, Dr Krishnamurthy does not think that is the reason why he has two series of patients where 10% had a psychotic reaction (on 250 mg twice a day). Perhaps the bioavailability of disulfiram manufactured locally is different from that available in Europe and the UK. Alternatively you could conceive of a genetic susceptibility to this particular effect.

BERGLUND
We changed the advice because reactions are so uncommon. The point is that if you have a very uncommon complication

and you advise GPs or psychiatrists that they could be contraindications, nobody dares to give psychiatric patients disulfiram That is a very strong influence. I think that this is a rare complication, according to the review and our data, and so it should be regarded simply as a rare complication and not as a contraindication to treatment with disulfiram.

CHICK
It's very important now that dual diagnosis is so fashionable.

LESCH
Can we agree that there is no absolute contraindication but that in these cases we should be cautious and use it in a low dosage?

CHICK
Thinking about your work, did you increase the dosage of disulfiram in your many patients to more than 400 mg?

LESCH
Never. We have never seen anything, so perhaps it is wise to say only 200 mg a day in these cases.

JOHNSEN
Discussing contraindications and so on and disulfiram in India and other places, the main use of disulfiram is in the rubber industry, so there is a lot of exposure to disulfiram. There is a very large production worldwide of this substance and there is another contraindication, which I think you should mention. That is rubber allergy, or other allergy to substances in rubber. This is not so infrequent in younger

males because they use condoms. Some of them are made of rubber and may cause skin symptoms or liver symptoms. I have seen both, so I think that's a contraindication that you should remember.

HARDT

I think that we should discuss combined treatment. Should acamprosate or naltrexone be used together with disulfiram and are there any other drugs that you feel could be used in combination with disulfiram?

LESCH

Besson et al[107] did a combined study and the sobriety rates were significantly increased combining acamprosate with disulfiram. We have used this combination occasionally in our centre for some years now and it seems to work well. We never combined disulfiram with naltrexone because we use naltrexone only as a damage limitation method, not as a sobriety measure. We have not seen any side effects.

CHICK

We still tend to use disulfiram as our first offer with regard to pharmacotherapy and of course some patients don't like the idea and refuse to take it. We can now prescribe acamprosate and obviously it has a different way of action but we have found it useful in people who like the disulfiram programme but keep on stopping it or forgetting to take it. We have had some good results by adding acamprosate. Patients say that

---

[107] Besson J, Aeby F, Kasas A *et al* Combined efficacy of acamprosate and disulfiram in the treatment of alcoholism: a controlled study. Alc Clin Exper Res 1998;22:573-579

they feel much happier and they continue to take the combination. We have done the same with naltrexone in that context, but we don't have so much experience.

BREWER

I agree that it can sometimes be a useful combination, rather like combined antidepressants. You don't use them if a single drug is effective, but if it's a resistant case, then you would think of combining them. What has impressed me about the two published studies, Besson et al and Carroll et al – one of which was randomised – is that disulfiram alone may be more effective than either naltrexone alone or acamprosate alone. I think that possibility needs to be made more widely known. Disulfiram is still the best drug we have, as shown by the research, but I think that it can usefully be combined with other drugs as well as with psychosocial treatments.

BERGLUND

This is a rather complicated question. We know, for example, that many patients receive several neuroleptics without any randomised studies indicating that it's useful. I think it's a great risk that people use several drugs at the same time without randomised controlled studies supporting this approach. We have this stratified study from Besson concerning acamprosate and disulfiram but it would be very good to use randomised studies with both drugs, before we issue recommendations on this point. I think SSRIs are a different story because SSRIs have no effect on drinking in my opinion but only on the depression of the alcoholic. So we treat one condition with SSRIs and the other with disulfiram. Another question concerns other deterrent drugs such as calcium carbimide [cyanamide]. It has a shorter half-life and more immediate effect. It has sometimes been recommended that it be used together with disulfiram in outpatient withdrawal. I don't know what your opinion about that is. I have been critical of this approach as well because we really have no controlled trials of the technique.

GEERLINGS

First I have also had good experiences with combination of other drugs with disulfiram. Mostly, patients choose one or other but sometimes it's best to use a combination. I agree that we need more and better randomised clinical trials to provide good evidence. However, our consensus and our clinical experience suggest that combinations have a place. It's the same with methadone. I think combined treatment is very important because opiate dependence has an odds ratio of more than 10 for alcoholism, so you have to treat it when it occurs. Sometimes the best treatment is one of these combinations, especially methadone and disulfiram. It is interesting but we do not have good experiences with calcium carbimide and it is now not easily available in the Netherlands.

POLDRUGO

I recently reviewed the literature on combined treatment. Our group has had experience with acamprosate and disulfiram showing a trend of improvement in the results but we don't have much data. The numbers were not big enough to do statistics. Then I found the work of Carroll et al[108] which is

---

[108] Carroll KM, Ziedonis D, O'Malley S *et al*. Pharmacologic interventions for abusers of alcohol and cocaine: a pilot study of

very interesting. This study was carried out in a small number of cocaine patients that is being replicated recently in a larger population group, also using psychotherapy.[109] So we now know how much and which type of psychotherapy you have to use and then there is the combination with naltrexone and disulfiram. I also found a very interesting but not very good paper on disulfiram and Gamma-hydroxybutyrate (GHB), a drug that is quite popular for alcoholism treatment in Italy. This improved the outcome as judged by the number of drinking days one year later. It seems this combination could be useful.

LESCH

Do we know anything about the interaction of disulfiram and GHB? It is a very good anti-withdrawal drug and it is also an anti-craving drug and is now available as tablets but I think its metabolism could be influenced by disulfiram. Do we know anything about that? I'd also like to make one comment about neuroleptics. I think there is now a neuroleptic being used to treat alcohol dependence. We have one Finnish trial together with the German group, where it is very clear that flupenthixol 10 mg daily for 14 days with disulfiram administration decreases the relapse rather significantly. It is difficult data to publish, so we make no

---

disulfiram versus naltrexone. *American Journal on the Addictions* 1993;2:77-79.

[109] This may be the study referred to: Carroll KM, Nich C, Ball SA, McCance E. Rounsavile B J. Treatment of cocaine and alcohol dependence with psychotherapy and disulfiram. Addiction 1998;93 (5), 713-728.

recommendation at present for the use of disulfiram with neuroleptic.

BERGLUND
The point I made earlier was about using several neuroleptics at the same time in schizophrenic patients, because this is a very common practice among psychiatrists, although there is no randomised study showing effectiveness. It wasn't really about neuroleptics in addiction.

BREWER
Just for the record, I have one patient at the moment who is on methadone, disulfiram and acamprosate. He had a very severe suicidal depressive illness that seemed to be related to opiate withdrawal. He seems to have no side effects on this combination.

JOHNSEN
I have some young patients who have been in France for one year. They have been on opiate substitution therapy with buprenorphine. What do you think of the possible combination with disulfiram? One of these patients has severe drinking problems too and we have to get control of his drinking problems because otherwise he will lose his substitution therapy, so could I combine it with disulfiram?

BREWER
Yes.

HARDT

I think that we are coming to the time when we are going to the restaurant in a few minutes, so if you still want to talk about disulfiram or other things, you can enjoy your wine at the same time. To sum up, I think those who've been here at the meeting have extensive clinical experience of disulfiram and find it useful. There are several ways in which it can be used but we all agree that it should be supervised and given for long periods, repeatedly if necessary. Its toxicity is well understood but not well known, so we must all try to teach our GPs how to use it properly but also to respect it. Disulfiram like all drugs can have adverse reactions. I think that it is too early to say much about combining it with other medication but it seems promising. The concept of keeping people abstinent with disulfiram and then trying to take craving away with another drug, requires further controlled clinical trials. We know all the difficulties involved in doing clinical trials on patients with alcohol problems.

I would like to thank you all. I think it is been a lively two hours and I hope that you will enjoy the rest of the evening.

POSTSCRIPT

The efficacy of disulfiram is also recognized by the World Health Organization.[110]

"Recommendation(s)

Acamprosate, disulfiram or naltrexone should be offered as part of treatment to reduce relapse to heavy alcohol use in alcohol dependent patients. The decision to use of acamprosate, disulfiram or naltrexone should be made taking into consideration patient preferences and availability.
Strength of recommendation: STRONG

Disulfiram should be offered to motivated patients in whom medication adherence can be monitored by treatment personnel, carers or family members, and when non-specialist health care providers are alert to potential adverse effects, including the disulfiram-alcohol reaction.
Strength of recommendation: STRONG"

(The quality of the evidence was not regarded as 'high' but it had not been updated since 2012)

---

[110] www.who.int/mental_health/mhgap/evidence/alcohol/q4/en/ accessed 29 May 2017

Chapter 9. INITIATING DISULFIRAM TREATMENT: some basic practices and principles

WHAT SORT OF PATIENT NEEDS DISULFIRAM?

Selection of patients for disulfiram treatment is not difficult. Many new patients may not need it at the outset of their treatment because, as already noted, apparently well motivated patients presenting for the first time and not facing serious risks to their domestic life, work, liberty or health, are likely to do well with minimal treatment. They should, however, have easy access to more focused treatment if necessary and that might include disulfiram. Conversely, patients with much failed treatment whose difficult situation is likely to become a lot worse if drinking is not immediately brought under control should be not only offered disulfiram but strongly encouraged to take it. In this sort of patient, failure to achieve immediate abstinence risks making the social and employment situation a lot worse and thus making the patient much more difficult to treat. Patients at high risk of the 'Five Ds' (divorce, dismissal, debt, de-housing and death) are patients who probably do need disulfiram and need it right away.

For the large number of patients in the middle of this spectrum, decisions about treatment do not necessarily have to be made in a hurry. The treatment menu of evidence-based interventions should be presented and discussed but if there is no great urgency – which often means: if the patients has already stopped drinking - some trial and error may be possible in the course of which both patient and therapist can decide on the most acceptable and least demanding treatment. Motivational interviewing may be particularly useful in this relatively relaxed situation. However, even if patients are not in serious danger of being thrown out of their job or home, a history of frequent relapses, especially if they have occurred despite treatment with acamprosate or naltrexone, should point very strongly in the direction of disulfiram, since it will maximise the effectiveness of other treatment components.

HOW QUICKLY CAN DISULFIRAM BE STARTED?

Formularies and even academic publications still often advise that disulfiram should not be started until at least 12 hours or in some cases 24 hours after the last drink. This advice is wrong, puts patients at high risk of continued alcohol abuse and has been completely illogical ever since it became easy to measure blood alcohol levels – i.e. for about the last 40 years. If, at the initial consultation, the reading on a breathalyser or saliva alcohol test-strip is zero or close to it, then disulfiram can be started either immediately or at the end of the consultation when all residual alcohol has disappeared. If it is not zero by then, a simple calculation - based on the finding that in most people, the blood alcohol level will fall by about 15 mg per 100ml per hour and often faster in seasoned drinkers - will indicate roughly how long the patient needs to remain in the clinic (and without access to alcohol) before disulfiram can be started. If the patient or his family (if any) do not think that he will be able to stop drinking for long enough to register zero, even with the help of family-supervised withdrawal medication, and particularly if there are present signs or a past history of at least moderately severe withdrawal symptoms, then a short admission will be necessary. Keeping in-patient treatment as short as possible is particularly important if personal preference or lack of NHS beds makes private treatment necessary but the patient is not among the small percentage of the UK population who have private insurance that also covers addiction treatment. Even a week in a private hospital will cost around £4500. The '28-day' programmes that are still popular with residential rehabs cost anything from £4500 to £20,000.

However, if there are no signs of withdrawal when the blood alcohol has fallen to 30 or 40 mg/100ml, it is very unlikely that more than overnight admission will be needed and disulfiram can be started either as soon as the breathalyser hits zero or first thing in the morning. There are several simple rating scales that quite accurately predict the likelihood of withdrawal symptoms severe enough to need hospital treatment.[111,112]

---

[111] Wetterling T, Weber B, Depfenhart M, Schneider B, Junghanns K. Development of a rating scale to predict the severity of alcohol withdrawal syndrome. Alcohol Alcohol. 2006 Nov-Dec;41(6):611-5
[112] Palmstierna T. A model for predicting alcohol withdrawal delirium. Psychiatr Serv. 2001 Jun;52(6):820-3.

WHAT SHOULD THE STARTING DOSE OF DISULFIRAM BE?

Until quite recently, the product information sheet in most countries advised that patients should take 800mg on Day1, 600mg on Day 2, 400mg on Day 3 and then 200mg daily. There is absolutely no rationale for this ancient and hallowed schedule if disulfiram is supervised and it risks antagonising the patient at a sensitive time if it leads to side effects that would not appear with a smaller dose. Since most patients will not risk drinking while taking disulfiram, 200 - 250mg – the usual amounts in a single tablet – is a reasonable starting dose, even though a significant proportion of patients would not get much or any reaction with alcohol on that dose. Some clinicians argue for a larger initial loading dose on the grounds that it may give an adequate DAR sooner than 200-250mg. They may have a case, especially for very challenging and ambivalent patients but the truth is that 60 years after disulfiram was introduced, we still do not know how quickly ALDH inhibition begins and how long it takes to reach its maximum. There is also an argument for starting on 150mg or even 100mg on the basis that side effects are less likely. However, alcoholics often talk to other alcoholics. Some patients will risk drinking and lower doses will inevitably mean that fewer of them will experience a DAR. If the word gets round that more than the occasional patient failed to get a significant DAR on those doses, more patients may be tempted to make the experiment. Even though, as previously discussed, most of them will persevere with treatment at a higher dose, some may suffer serious social or legal consequences (including imprisonment) before the dose reaches the right level. For patients who are not in such delicate situations and where achieving immediate abstinence and maintaining it is not essential, the level of the starting dose is less important than acceptance of the principle that if continued drinking makes it necessary, the dose must be increased. As noted elsewhere, not all prescribers do accept it but it seems to us a very logical position.

As we have seen, some patients need doses of 600mg daily[113] or more before they stop drinking.[114, 115] It is not sufficiently recognised that disulfiram is a *pro-drug* and needs to be converted to its active metabolite. In a few patients, this conversion may be inefficient for various reasons, possibly including serious liver disease.[116] Furthermore, differences in the manufacturing process can have significant effects on the bioavailability of disulfiram, which may thus vary from country to country.[117]

---

[113] Brewer C. Long-term, high-dose disulfiram in the treatment of alcohol abuse. *Br J Psychiat* 1993;163:687-9.

[114] Newton-Howes G, Levack WM, McBride S, Gilmor M, Tester R. Non-physiological mechanisms influencing disulfiram treatment of alcohol use disorder: A grounded theory study. Drug Alc Depend 2016;165:126-31.

[115] Bickel WK, Rizzuto P, Zielony RD, Klobas J, Pangiosonlis P, Mernit R, Knight WF. Combined Behavioral and Pharmacological Treatment of Alcoholic Methadone Patients. J Subst Abuse. 1988-1989;1(2):161-71.

[116] Johansson B. A review of the pharmacokinetics and pharmacodynamics of disulfiram and its metabolites. Acta Psychiatr Scand Suppl. 1992;369:15-26.

[117] Andersen MP. Lack of bioequivalence between disulfiram formulations. Exemplified by a tablet/effervescent tablet study. Acta Psychiatr Scand Suppl. 1992;369:31-5.

IN-PATIENT DETOXIFICATION

If getting consent to treatment is difficult because withdrawal symptoms need high doses of sedating medication to control them, or if the patient is incoherent or delirious, the first dose of disulfiram can wait until the worst is over, usually after no more than 3 to 4 days. If the patient's family are able to cope with him back home at that stage, he can be discharged, if necessary with a limited supply of benzodiazepines or other anti-withdrawal medication to be kept in the care of the family and tailed off over the next few days.

Attitudes to prescribing hypnotics for more than a very short period (or at all) have hardened in the last decade or two but in the first week or two after withdrawal, when the patient may be feeling both physically and emotionally unwell, having to stay awake and contemplate past excesses and deficiencies may not be helpful and there is a case for saying that chemical sleep is better than no sleep. Since initial insomnia tends to be commoner than early waking, a very short-acting hypnotic, designed to get the patient to sleep but with no or minimal hangover effect in the morning, may be the logical choice. In some countries, oral midazolam is a standard hypnotic and is very suitable for this purpose, since its elimination half-life is typically about two hours.

We all have our preferences about the management of withdrawal and provided that the preferred regime protects the patient against *delirium tremens* and withdrawal fits, and gives him a reasonable night's sleep while he is in hospital, the precise pharmacological details are not very important.

The benzodiazepine loading technique, in which increasing doses of diazepam or lorazepam are given as symptoms increase, to a level where the patient is reasonably comfortable or even a little sleepy, has much to commend it. Top-up doses can be repeated as needed. There is no need to prescribe specific anticonvulsants except for patients with established epilepsy, who should be taking them anyway. Anti-psychotic drugs should *never* be used prophylactically and rarely, if ever, in established delirium. They increase the risk of seizures, do not prevent the onset of hallucinations and can inflict unpleasant side-effects on patients who already have several unpleasant symptoms. In private practice and if cost is unimportant, higher sedative doses can be combined with having an attendant in the room to make sure the patient doesn't fall if he gets out of bed. Diazepam and lorazepam have the advantage that both are available for parenteral administration, which is sometimes needed. One of my patients was still very tremulous and uncomfortable despite several 20mg doses of oral diazepam. After 70mg of diazepam slowly infused intravenously over the next 20 minutes, she felt much better but was still talking animatedly and coherently. Rarely, patients are unresponsive to benzodiazepines. Even today, d*elirium tremens* is sometimes lethal, especially for patients in poor health from other alcohol-related conditions. Sometimes, admission to an intensive care unit is needed; very occasionally, patients need to be intubated.

A comfortable and attentive detox helps to get the doctor-patient relationship off to a good start, especially if previous withdrawals have been unhappy experiences. Unless there is really nowhere else for them to go, very few physically-dependent patients need to be in hospital for more than five days and many can be discharged after three or four. Even homeless patients can be transferred to a hostel in a few days unless there are pressing medical (or, more rarely, psychiatric) reasons for them to occupy an acute hospital bed. Most patients with a job should be able to return to work within two weeks at most and often within a week. In other cases, some sort of day patient programme may be indicated but outpatient visits once or twice a week initially may be adequate. While the patient is in hospital or, if admission is not indicated, during the few days after the initial consultation, a disulfiram supervisor should have been identified, agreed, and trained. If no supervisor is immediately available, supervision should be done as a day-patient or as an out-patient, or through home visits from a community nurse, but particularly if the patient is keen to return to work, the outpatient visit need not involve much more than seeing a nurse or pharmacist to receive a dose of disulfiram. If necessary, patients can visit the ward daily during the first week but as noted earlier, Monday/Wednesday/Friday or even Monday/Thursday dosing with group or individual counselling sessions as needed will usually work well. In a thrice-weekly schedule, it is usual to give double the daily dose on Mondays and Wednesdays and triple on Fridays, though disulfiram's prolonged action means that for the majority of patients, this may have more symbolic than pharmacological significance.

INVESTIGATIONS AND WHEN TO DO THEM.

In the absence of obvious contra-indications discovered during history-taking and physical examination (which are few and nearly all relative rather than absolute) there is no need to wait for the results of blood tests or ECGs before starting disulfiram. It is usual to request standard LFTs, haematology and electrolytes but whatever alcohol-related abnormalities may be found, they will usually improve very quickly once drinking stops. Patients should be warned about possible side-effects and how to recognise them, as discussed in Ch. 14, and the potentially fatal risks of the DAR, but although it is useful and desirable to have baseline readings, there is no need for frequent blood tests unless there is an obvious medical indication for them. For example, a patient with significant anaemia should probably be retested in a few days in case there has been some gastro-intestinal bleeding but elevated liver function tests can usually wait for a week or two before being repeated. Obviously, any acute medical or surgical condition – alcohol-related or otherwise – should receive appropriate treatment. The special investigative requirements of patients who will clearly need a court report are covered in Ch. 13.

PSYCHOTROPIC MEDICATION – ANTIDEPRESSANTS, ANTIPSYCHOTICS, MOOD STABILISERS.

Unless a patient is already taking antidepressant or, more rarely, antipsychotic drugs, *and is taking them for good reasons*, there is virtually never any indication for starting them until the patient has been abstinent for several weeks and even the need for continuing medication should be questioned. This is because much of what is called depression and anxiety or 'dual diagnosis' in people who are drinking heavily is the *result* of their drinking and its unhappy consequences and not the cause of it. [118] Alternatively, it may be an independent and unrelated event.[119] After a few weeks of sobriety, they are likely to be feeling very much better. If they have been taking antidepressants during this period of improvement, both the patient and the doctor may be tempted to conclude that the improvement is due to the antidepressants rather than just to the passage of time, abstinence from alcohol and regression to the mean. If a patient is still significantly depressed or anxious after a month or two of abstinence and not obviously improving, then a careful assessment can be made of the need for further treatment, which may or may not include the pharmacological kind.

Another reason for caution in antidepressant prescribing is the increasing evidence that for most patients who receive them, they have little or no specific effect, as opposed to the considerable – and widely underestimated - placebo and non-specific effects that are responsible for the majority of the improvement in most placebo-controlled trials, particularly the most rigorous and high-quality ones. Furthermore,

---

[118] Davidson K. Diagnosis of depression in alcohol dependence: changes in prevalence with drinking status. Brit J Psychiat 1993;166, 199-204.

[119] Farmer RF, Seeley JR, Kosty DB, et al. No reliable evidence that emotional disorders are proximal antecedents, concomitants, or short-term consequences of first episode alcohol use disorders in a representative community sample. J Stud Alc Drugs, 78(2), 222–231 (2017).

examples of dishonest reporting, serious conflicts of interest and 'data massage' in industry-sponsored publications are not rare, exemplified by one trial in which "serious irregularities in the statistical analysis of the results... turned a study with essentially negative findings into a paper that was used to promote the widespread use of a treatment that had at most a marginal and questionable value".[120] It is increasingly clear that a significant advantage for antidepressants over placebo is largely restricted to patients who are severely depressed.[121] "Drug-placebo differences...became large enough to be clinically important only in the very small minority of patient populations with severe major depression".[122] They may also have useful specific effects in patients whose depression does not seem to be related to adverse life-events or unhelpful cognitive, behavioural or personality characteristics. Most alcoholics cannot easily be fitted into that description and their 'depression' is often synonymous with 'understandable misery'.

I can recall only a single patient (no longer living) for whom starting psychotropic medication in the first few days after admission was both indicated and justified by subsequent

---

[120] Le Noury J et al. Restoring Study 329: efficacy and harms of paroxetine and imipramine in treatment of major depression in adolescence. BMJ 2015;351:h4320

[121] Thase ME, Larsen KG, Kennedy SH. Assessing the 'true' effect of active antidepressant therapy v. placebo in major depressive disorder: use of a mixture model Brit J Psychiat .2011, 199 (6) 501-507

[122] Ioannidis JP. Effectiveness of antidepressants: an evidence myth constructed from a thousand randomized trials? Philos Ethics Humanit Med. 2008 May 27;3:14.

events. He was an alcoholic clergyman with a double first in divinity from Oxford who had been forced by alcoholism to resign from his parish.

It had been suspected that he was manic-depressive but he had never stayed abstinent for long enough for anybody to be reasonably sure and nobody had given him a trial of mood-stabilisers. Once he had recovered from withdrawal and started taking disulfiram for the first time, he had his first dose of lithium. About three days later, he said that a feeling of peace descended on him that he had not known for many years. He remained abstinent thereafter and took lithium regularly. [123]

---

[123] His rather classy rehabilitation took place in the library of Lambeth Palace (conveniently just across the Thames from my alcoholism clinic at Westminster Hospital) where he was given the job of rearranging and cataloguing books that dated, in some cases, from Henry VIII's break with Rome in 1536 and earlier. He was not far off retiring age and when he did eventually retire two or three years later, he invited me in my clinical capacity to a farewell dinner in the Great Hall that had been arranged by the then Archbishop of Canterbury, Robert Runcie.

Chapter 10. SUPERVISION IN THE CONTEXT OF PROBATION AND PAROLE
Dealing with recurrent alcoholic offenders.

Although Ruth Fox seems to have been the first author to argue, in 1955, that supervision of disulfiram was essential to maximising success in everyday, voluntary alcoholism treatment, the first study in which disulfiram was routinely supervised was not published until over a decade later.[124] Peter Bourne and his colleagues began their paper: "During the last several years, about 50,000 arrests have been made annually for public intoxication in the City of Atlanta". The city's population at the time was about one million. After noting the "obviously inadequate facilities for helping these people" and the "tremendous economic burden they represent", they describe how the Department of Psychiatry at a prestigious local university was asked (and presumably funded) by the City administration to do a year-long study and come up with a Plan. Commendably, instead of a confident and unitary City-wide campaign, they decided on a few small pilot studies, one of which involved offering supervised disulfiram "free and voluntarily to those who appeared in court charged with public intoxication". Not many of them accepted but in those who did, "the subsequent success of [disulfiram] in keeping them abstinent was impressive. Some of those most spectacularly helped had

---

[124] Bourne PG, Alford JA. Bowcock JZ. Treatment of skid-row alcoholics with Disulfiram Quart J Stud Alc 1966;27:42-.48.

been seen innumerable times" by the courts who "believed they had very little potential for sustained abstinence".

Thus encouraged, and in what might be regarded as a logical development, the team - or perhaps the courts - suggested offering selected offenders the chance to accept a suspended sentence, "provided they agreed to take disulfiram under supervision daily".[125] They could thus compare voluntary vs "semi-compulsory" treatment in a group notorious for expressing good intentions that they are "rarely able to maintain." In the pilot study, family members were usually recruited as supervisors. In the second study, most of the offenders were recurrent 'skid-row' alcoholics who had lost contact with any supportive family members they might once have had and the supervision was done by probation officers at the court. Although the study was uncontrolled, the results were truly impressive, given that virtually all the 132 patients recruited during a four-month period had long histories of severe alcohol abuse resistant to other methods of treatment. A particularly notable and encouraging finding was that 61 were still taking disulfiram at the end of the 9-month study period, even though their suspended sentences had long expired. Among the most "spectacular" individual outcomes were "several patients who had served as much as 10 years in jail…in consecutive 30-day [drunkenness] sentences". On disulfiram, they had managed to stay dry for several months when the study ended and had "been able to hold down steady jobs during this time".

---

[125] This idea had actually been floated by Martensen-Larsen in 1949 but not formally studied.

Another 17 had at least taken disulfiram throughout the agreed 30-60 days but however long they abstained, all patients were encouraged to take advantage of their sobriety by joining AA, "various religious groups, and whatever psychiatric facilities were available". The local department of Labour actively helped with job-finding and patients were also referred for treatment of their presumably quite numerous medical conditions. This effective and humane programme worked well even though it catered almost exclusively for "the lowest stratum" of alcoholic patients – the sort ignored or rejected by many services as "having too low a yield of success" for anyone to bother trying to treat. Before we look at some possible reasons for the neglect of both probation-linked disulfiram and this numerically important group of patients with large social costs who might benefit greatly from it, let us examine some possible objections.

If, as some clinicians insist, disulfiram has a high incidence of Adverse Events (AEs), one would expect to see evidence of its toxicity and dangers in this sizeable cohort of generally malnourished, underclass and quite often homeless 'Skid Row' alcoholics with "extremely poor general health". Only patients who were overtly psychotic or had a history of myocardial infarction were excluded. There was a single case of dermatitis (which is usually mild, localised and self-limiting, as discussed in Ch.14) but not one serious AE was reported, "either from taking [disulfiram] or experiencing the reaction with alcohol".

The number of patients in the probation-linked group who risked drinking on disulfiram is not stated but of the pilot study's 64 patients who started on disulfiram, 16 tried to drink and "experienced a reaction". There are no details about the severity of the reaction but those who experienced it generally "adhered closely...and were in many ways the most successful patients". If, as implied, all or most of this 'testing-out' group had a sufficiently impressive and deterrent reaction, that may have been because the disulfiram dosage in both studies was 500mg daily. That there were so few AEs in this very high-compliance group taking this comparatively high dose is further testimony to the safety of disulfiram compared with unchecked alcoholism; and to the serious exaggeration of its dangers by many critics.

An indication of the lethal dangers faced even now by untreated or inappropriately treated 'skid row' alcoholics comes from a series of 42 post-mortems on alcoholics mainly from economically deprived and Latino backgrounds who died in unlicensed treatment facilities in Los Angeles between 2003 and 2014.[126] (The authors believe that similar problems exist in other areas of the USA with large Latino populations.) Most were young or middle-aged and only three were 60 or over. Six died from *delirium tremens,* 11 from acute alcohol poisoning, another 11 from medical complications of chronic alcoholism and three from diabetes – which may also be one of those complications. In three

---

[126] Su K-C, Nguyen L, Rogers C. Deaths in Unlicensed Alcohol Rehabilitation Facilities. J Forensic Sci, January 2017, Vol. 62, No. 1 doi: 10.1111/1556-4029.13253

cases, the treatment of the patient was so incompetent and inappropriate that the death was considered a homicide.[127]

Bourne et al came to the restrained and surely justifiable conclusion that for some alcoholic offenders at least, probation-linked disulfiram "has tremendous potential". They also noted that it was very much cheaper than repeated arrests and court appearances, even if offenders avoided the additional public expense of a prison sentence. Having a significant period of abstinence for perhaps the first time in many years enabled some offenders to "get a start on a new way of life". Finally, they made what should be a rather obvious point that if supervised disulfiram works so well in this very damaged and discouraging group of patients, it might work even better with the much less damaged and much more promising alcoholics who comprise the majority of patients in nearly all alcoholism services and clinics, both private and public.

Other American researchers had similar ideas – and similarly impressive outcomes. Liebson and Faillace[128] described an ingenious method of improving compliance in another group of 10 poor prognosis skid-row alcoholics. Disulfiram was

---

[127] In one of these 'culturally sensitive' facilities ("all decedents were Spanish-speaking men with severe alcoholism") the standard treatment for DTs included such fruits of ancient cultural wisdom as "plac[ing] cut onion or garlic near [the] nose".
[128] Liebson I, Faillace LA. The pharmacological reinforcement of disulfiram maintenance in chronic alcoholism. *NIDA Research Monograph* 1971 pp 1266-1273

combined in a capsule with chlordiazepoxide[129] in doses of 75 – 125mg daily. The idea was that the sedative-tranquillising effect would act as a positive reinforcer, which would be an incentive for patients to continue taking disulfiram, rather as in a later study [130] that combined disulfiram with methadone maintenance therapy, described in Ch. 13. Depending on the time of administration, the chlordiazepoxide would act as either a tranquilliser or a hypnotic – effects that would be attractive to many alcoholics and much less damaging than using alcohol for these purposes. Weekly supervision is implied, though not entirely clear, but improving compliance was clearly central to the study. The patients had probably all committed numerous alcohol-related offences but their treatment was not a condition of probation or parole. This was a pilot study but six of the ten patients had remained in treatment for a mean of six months at the time of the report.

A retrospective study in Colorado Springs (population c. 250,000 at the time) investigated the effectiveness of supervised disulfiram for 12 months as one condition of a probation order in recurrent "revolving door" alcoholic offenders.[131] Some patients left town, often for legitimate

---

[129] Note for non-medics. Chlordiazepoxide was one of the first benzodiazepine sedatives, widely known by its commercial name Librium. 25mg three times daily was a fairly standard dose but alcoholics often have high tolerance for tranquillisers as well as for alcohol.
[130] Liebson I, Bigelow G, Flame J. Alcoholism among methadone patients: a specific treatment method. *Amer J Psychiat* 1973;130:483-485
[131] Haynes SN. Contingency management in a municipally administered Antabuse program for alcoholics. J Behaviour Therapy Exper Psychiat 1973;4:31-32.

reasons, and 12% were jailed for non-compliance but in the remainder, acting as their own controls, the study found *an almost 13-fold reduction in alcohol-related offences* [our italics] compared with their previous record. As with the Atlanta study, the long history of recurrent and frequent offending meant that patients could reasonably act as their own controls, yet these impressive results were achieved despite only twice weekly dosage at the probation office.

The first British patient I treated with disulfiram as one condition of a probation order was not like Atlanta's homeless, wretched-of-the-earth, habitual public drunkards but the son of a family of minor Scottish aristocrats who lived on his own in a mews house that stood out because of its grubby and peeling paintwork in a smart residential area just round the corner from Harrods. I forget the nature of Stuart's latest crime but he had often come before the local magistrates court, just across Horseferry Road from my clinic at the Westminster Hospital and his probation officer thought it unlikely that he could dissuade the magistrates from making good their several previous and increasingly tetchy warnings that aristo or not, they would send him to prison if he didn't mend his ways. His solicitor, who had asked for a psychiatric report more in desperation than expectation, thought that this time, a prison sentence was certain and merely hoped that my report might help to reduce its length. Stuart was not a daily drinker and had been alcohol-free for several days when first seen. His problem – a common one – was drunken binges every few weeks during which he left a trail of damaged property, bodies, feelings and relationships.

He was an obvious and pressing candidate for supervised disulfiram (and for a challenge dose of alcohol to make sure that the dose was adequate: no second bite of the therapeutic and pharmacological cherry here) but who would or could do the supervising? Not Stuart's estranged family, who sent his remittance on condition that he left them alone. Not his two very-much-ex-wives, his very few and currently outraged non-alcoholic friends or the slightly more numerous alcoholic ones. It did not occur to me to ask the probation officer himself if he would be the supervisor, partly because I had not then come across the paper by Peter Bourne and his colleagues in distant Atlanta but also because I did not meet Stuart's probation officer until a few weeks later. In those pre-internet days – this was about 1980 – getting hold of papers from relatively minor specialist journals, or even hearing about them and reading the abstracts, was not straightforward, especially if the paper had been published many years previously.[132]

Tribalism, urban geography, the British army's Special Air Service and religion provided the solution. Even when sober, Stuart spent little time dwelling on religious thoughts but on his sober or repentant Sundays, he was sufficiently tribal and Scottish to attend services at St Columba's, the elegant 1950s Grade II-listed Church of Scotland building that is also just round the corner from Harrods. It was Stuart himself who suggested that the man in charge of the place might agree to supervise the disulfiram and he was right. The dominie was a

---

[132] In 1966, there were only two NHS specialists in England dealing exclusively with alcoholics. I'm not sure about Scotland or Wales.

friendly and sympathetic cleric and more than happy to do his bit to save Stuart's soul (and body) from a very real demon. He was also about as no-nonsense a supervisor as anyone – including the magistrates - could have wished. The Rev Fraser McLuskey MC,[133] had become famous during the war as the unarmed 'parachute padre' who brought the comforts of religion to SAS units parachuted into France just before D-Day. I knew, and Stuart knew, that he would quickly and unfailingly let us know if Stuart didn't turn up for his daily dose and we could rely on him to appoint and instruct a trustworthy vicarial substitute if he were out of town. After some discussion, the magistrates agreed that Stuart could avoid prison if he complied with daily disulfiram and, of course, avoided further offences for the next year. Both of which he did.

Impressed with the unexpected double success of both keeping Stuart out of prison and keeping him sober for an unprecedented period, John Smith, his probation officer, came to see me to discuss using the same technique with some of his numerous other alcoholic old lags. Many of them were of no fixed abode – an ancient phrase still much used today – and lived in the Church Army and Salvation Army hostels round the corner not from Harrods but from Victoria Station, where even more desperate homeless alcoholics spent the night in the stationary trains. However, most of John's alcoholic probationers had homes and often wives and children as well. Quite a few had jobs.

---

[133] Military Cross.

That was how the Westminster probation-linked disulfiram programme came about and evolved. At first, John – and later, his probation colleagues – supervised the disulfiram on Mondays, Wednesdays and Fridays, usually combining it with an ordinary counselling session. As most of the patients stayed dry, or had only brief lapses of compliance that were quickly aborted, they had progressively fewer problems for which they needed counselling, so the task of supervision was delegated, after a very short training session, to the receptionists, who dissolved the disulfiram, saw that it was followed by a second glass of water, and put a tick against the patient's name in the register. If there was a cross rather than a tick, the probation officer would investigate and if necessary, remind the offender that both attending the office and swallowing disulfiram were conditions that he had agreed to as part of the probationary bargain. If he wanted to renegotiate that bargain, the magistrates would be happy to accommodate him the next or even the same day. If not, he needed to get back in line, and quickly.

The terms of the bargain were actually more flexible than they might seem. What the patient agreed to, and the magistrates accepted, was that he would have treatment as directed by me, it being understood that that treatment would include disulfiram. However, if disulfiram had to be discontinued because of serious side-effects, for example, he would not automatically be in breach of probation. That never happened but if it had, it would have been possible at that time to change the medication to cyanamide without getting a new probation order, though the probation service might have sought the views of the magistrates about the change. Today, the alternative might be tagging with one of the high-tech devices that quickly detect, record and – in some cases – transmit by radio to a central monitoring post – any use of alcohol, as discussed shortly.

It was while seriously searching the published literature on disulfiram for the first time in order to write our paper that we came across the paper by Bourne et al. Our results, published in the BMJ in 1983, were, as we wrote: "at least as encouraging as those reported by Bourne et al and Haynes. Only three of our 16 patients [19%] consistently refused to [continue taking] disulfiram compared with 46% of [Bourne's] and [37%] of Haynes's". One of those three, after being briefly imprisoned for the breach of probation, resumed disulfiram after his release. Our average abstinence of 30 weeks compared with 12 weeks for Bourne's patients.[134] We also found that offenders "generally required less probation work than if they had continued drinking and offending" and that as in Atlanta, "several patients asked for their disulfiram to be continued after the probation order expired". It is both interesting and clinically important that while only a quarter of the Atlanta patients risked drinking while taking disulfiram, just over half of ours did. This underlines both the challenging and 'difficult' features of recurrent alcoholic offenders and the need for dose increases where the DAR is inadequate. However, the fact that none of our probationers was charged with an offence while

---

[134] Brewer C, Smith J. Probation-linked supervised disulfiram in the treatment of habitual drunken offenders: results of a pilot study. BMJ. 1983;287:1282-83.

abstaining suggests that their offending was generally due to their alcoholism rather than to fundamentally criminal attitudes.

A similar approach to heroin-related crime was made possible when naltrexone became available in Britain in 1985 and was offered to a few Westminster offenders. A study in the US had shown that just as alcoholic offenders became much easier to manage with disulfiram, it was possible for imprisoned but detoxified heroin addicts who took naltrexone under supervision to leave prison for day-release work programmes without the high rates of relapse that were the rule without the protection that naltrexone provided.[135] On the naltrexone programme, heroin addicts, previously regarded as occupying a low position on the prison's "trust ladder" quickly became regarded as some of the more reliable inmates. Much more impressive were two controlled studies – from Singapore and the US - where the benefit was shown in heroin-related offenders on parole or probation and living in their usual environment with its usual stresses and temptations. In the Singapore study, patients took oral naltrexone thrice weekly after work under close supervision at a building immediately (and symbolically) adjacent to Changi Prison, where they also gave supervised urine samples. A year later, 75% were still opiate-free, compared with 25% in the identical programme before naltrexone was

---

[135] Brahen L, Henderson R, Capone T. Naltrexone treatment in a jail work-release program. J. Clin. Psychol. 1984;45, 49-52.

added.[136] In the US study, the results in the naltrexone group were very clearly superior to naltrexone-free treatment, even though dosing was only twice weekly.[137]

DETERRENCE BY RAPID DETECTION OF DRINKING AND INSTANT SANCTIONS.

The alcohol-detecting tags briefly mentioned earlier have given promising results in a study done in Dakota[138] but are much more intrusive than disulfiram. Judges impose a special set of conditions on repeat drink-driving offenders, requiring them to submit to morning and evening alcohol testing as a condition of bail and, in many cases, freedom to continue driving. Alternatively, they must wear an alcohol-detecting and recording ankle tag that can be examined frequently. Evidence of drinking or a missed test constitute a violation of bond, parole or probation arrangements, which may be immediately revoked, usually leading to immediate 24-hour imprisonment and driving licence withdrawal. Interestingly – and in accord with our argument about the importance of deterrence – these positive results are consistent with the finding that average-speed cameras have more effect than

---

[136] Chan KY. The Singapore naltrexone community-based project for heroin addicts compared with drugfree community-based program: the first cohort. J Clin Med 1996;3:87-92

[137] Cornish JW, Metzger D, Woody GW et al. Naltrexone pharmacotherapy for opioid dependent federal probationers. J Subs Abuse Treat 1997;14:529-534

[138] Loudenburg R, Drube G, Leonardson G. South Dakota 24/7 Sobriety Program Evaluation Findings Report. Dakota: Mountain Plains Evaluation, LLC. 2010

increased penalties on both speed and speeding, presumably because of the near certainty of detection.[139]

Given the large problem of alcohol-related crime, our encouraging results, their similarity to the results of other published studies and their publication in Britain's most widely read medical journal, it is reasonable to wonder why programmes like those that evolved in Westminster are so rare in Britain. The reasons for the lack of interest by senior British addiction academics in probation-linked pharmacological treatments for addiction-related crime are political rather than medical and are discussed in an Appendix that can be accessed on the book's website at planetservetus.org.

---

[139] Linssen J. Personal communication and paper presented at the Intelligent Traffic System Association of Malaysia Congress, Kuala Lumpur, Feb 21-23 2017

Chapter 11. HOW DISULFIRAM FACILITATES PSYCHOSOCIAL INTERVENTIONS AND REHABILITATION: the language-learning analogy, the OLITA programme, and its 9-year follow-up

Many of the most challenging alcoholic patients never acquired more than basic social and employment skills, if that, and often have to deal with life problems that began in childhood or even *in utero*.[140] However, for most services and clinicians, they are a much smaller group than patients whose contact with the world of work is less intermittent and tenuous. This larger group may need some help with basic social and employment skills but most of them have worked, still have social relationships and are employable or employed.

Nevertheless, any specific benefits of treatment will be reduced or completely nullified if they regularly fail to turn up for planned treatment, or do appear but are too drunk or hungover to absorb and retain much information. Incorporating supervised disulfiram into such programmes greatly increases the likelihood that patients will both turn up for their appointments and benefit from them.

---

[140] Apart from foetal alcohol syndrome and the psychological and emotional consequences of poor parenting, the children of alcoholics may also have an increased risk of brain damage in infancy, childhood and adolescence due to poor cooperation with obstetric and neonatal care, non-accidental injury and more frequent fights than the children of more promising and nurturing families.

In the 1980s, this was demonstrated in one prospective study by Sereny et al mentioned earlier.[141] Noting that a significant number of their patients relapsed repeatedly despite complying well with a good conventional out-patient treatment programme, they devised a radical but constructive response after three relapses. Instead of declining to offer further treatment, they told patients that they could return for treatment, or remain in it, but only if they agreed to take disulfiram under professional supervision during their outpatient attendance. 68 of 73 patients agreed to this arrangement.

'Total success' was defined as being sober for at least six months and remaining in the supervised disulfiram program at the time of assessment, or having been discharged from supervised disulfiram after 12 months of sobriety. By these criteria, 40% of patients were totally successful and 18% were partially successful. Only 29% were failures and 13% had not been in treatment for long enough to be categorised. Those are good results in a group of patients who by definition would normally be regarded as having a poor prognosis and would often be refused further treatment. In other respects, their management appears to have been similar to that during their previous treatment episodes. OLITA (Outpatient Long-term Intensive Therapy for Alcoholics) is a version of this programme that extended over two years and produced even better results despite even more challenging patients. The results were maintained for

---

[141] Sereny G, Sharma V, Holt J, Gordis E. Mandatory supervised Antabuse therapy in an out-patient alcoholism program: a study. Alc Clin Exper Res 1986;10:290-292.

what is, by the standards of clinical trials, a remarkable and record-breaking nine-year period of follow-up. We shall return to it shortly.

The process of helping patients to learn certain skills and to practise them for long enough to be reasonably confident, competent and automatic in their performance, is what in other contexts we call 'education' or 'training'. As clinicians who learned a second language for reasons of work or travel, it occurred to us that effective treatment of alcoholics and heroin addicts was also an *educational* process. We argued that it had many similarities with the ways in which people learn (or fail to learn) a second language and that the analogy had important practical implications for alcoholism treatment.[142]

Any English-speaker who has tried to learn a foreign language knows how many obstacles there are to achieving fluency. Initially, one continues to think in English and each individual word has to be mentally translated. Many people give up at this stage, or satisfy themselves with a few basic words or phrases. It is so much easier not to bother and to hope (not always in vain) that if you speak English loudly and slowly, foreigners will understand. When you have thought, spoken, cursed, joked, written and dreamed exclusively in English all your life, it can be hard for those

---

[142] Brewer C, Streel E. Learning the language of abstinence in addiction treatment: some similarities between relapse-prevention with disulfiram, naltrexone and other pharmacological antagonists and intensive 'immersion' methods of foreign language teaching. Substance Abuse, 2003; 24(3) 157-173.

without special linguistic aptitudes to change. Similar difficulties confront alcoholics and other substance abusers trying to change their habits.

Because learning foreign languages is an important area of education, there has been much research into which methods are efficient and cost-effective and, equally important, which methods are not. Essentially, there are two approaches to language teaching. Primary and secondary schools often use a 'drip-feed' approach in which students with varying degrees of motivation are taught in a fairly passive way for short periods once or twice a week. What they do between classes with the skills and information they acquire is left very much to them. Inevitably, many will hardly give it a thought from one lesson to the next. Many out-patient alcoholism programmes have similar limitations. Pupils/patients may be genuinely keen to learn but if they don't see results quickly, disillusionment, boredom or demoralisation may set in.

The other approach regards intensive exposure or 'immersion' as the norm and sees non-intensive, 'drip-feed' exposure as an inefficient use of teaching resources. Intensive, all-day immersion enables a class of adults to learn Italian up to the equivalent of Grade A in the GCSE school-leaving exam in only 80 hours spread over two weeks, compared with five years for the normal school Italian syllabus. Like the difference between treatment with and without disulfiram, this difference has much more than mere statistical '$p<0.05$' significance. Furthermore, immersion methods make the educational/counselling process easier for the teacher/clinician as well as the student/patient.

Living in a foreign country for several months (and not spending much time with one's compatriots) is an effective informal way of learning a new language and its cultural associations. Language teachers call this 'submersion'. The superiority of 'immersion' and 'submersion' methods also explains why they are favoured in most private language schools. They combine *cue exposure* (i.e. students are exposed to a situation that requires them to have a conversation) with *response-prevention* (i.e. the students are prevented from conversing *in English*). Any clinician familiar with the techniques or even the principles of Cognitive-Behavioural Therapy will recognise this combination of Exposure and Response-Prevention (ERP) as a standard, evidence-based treatment for changing responses and behaviour that are agreed by both patient and therapist to be unhelpful (or 'maladaptive'). ERP helps spider-phobic patients to get used to spiders instead of fleeing from them. It enables agoraphobic patients to leave their houses. It helps obsessive-compulsive patients spend less time on their rituals. High fees are charged for intensive language courses, using these principles, that enable students to achieve useful levels of fluency in as little as one week. For most purposes, it is more important and useful to have the confidence to converse in a foreign language, even if imperfectly than to have a good theoretical knowledge of vocabulary and grammar but lack the confidence to use it.

ANALOGIES WITH THE TREATMENT OF ALCOHOLISM

The equivalent of immersion or submersion in treatment for alcoholism would require prolonged and repeated cue-exposure to real-life situations involving alcohol, or associated with it, while response-prevention provided a barrier to the actual consumption of alcohol. It would encourage the notions (or cognitions) that not using alcohol - like not habitually speaking English - is compatible with a reasonably satisfying existence; that there are other ways of dealing with anxieties and sorrows than by drowning them; and that temptation is not irresistible

Some alcoholism treatment programmes do emphasise cue-exposure to alcohol, even providing pseudo-bars in which to practise abstinence in the presence of pseudo-temptation. They also encourage the practice of alternative behaviours that do not involve using alcohol.[143] These range from drinking alcohol-free beverages (and becoming assertive enough to demand them), through anxiety management to joining evening classes in order to get a new set of friends. Unfortunately, these programmes are much closer to the 'drip feed' model of education than to 'immersion' techniques. The counselling and group or individual therapy (the teaching) and the supervised exposure to real-life or, more commonly, simulated cues and temptations (the practice) will rarely last more than an hour or two at a time. The same is

---

[143] As explained in Ch. 18, a similar process helps opiate addicts treated with depot or implanted naltrexone to get used to walking past - rather than into - the houses where their dealers live and to refuse seductive offers of heroin from their still-using friends.)

true of AA meetings. Hodgson emphasises "..the importance of practising coping skills when facing temptation and not just in the peace and quiet of the therapist's office".[144] That is precisely what disulfiram makes it much easier for patients to do. And as with language, having the confidence to use coping skills unhesitatingly and automatically, even if imperfectly, is more important than knowing what to do in theory but not being able to use that knowledge when it is most needed.

Patients in most treatment programmes leave the artificial atmosphere of the out-patient clinic or rehab to enter a world where it is very easy to escape from the discipline of treatment and to forget or fluff the coping techniques. Many soon revert to old habits, often unthinkingly, and the temptation to do so is rarely absent. If drinking does occur, the 'abstinence violation effect' often combines with the effects of intoxication to increase the risk that the relapse will be a serious one. Even minor relapses may undermine the patient's self-esteem and belief in his ability to change. Exposure to cues involving alcohol is the daily experience of alcoholics living in the real world. Disulfiram provides the response-prevention that is particularly important in the first few weeks and months of treatment if those new coping skills are to have the best chance of becoming established.

---

[144] Hodgson R. Resisting temptation: a psychological analysis. Brit J Addict. 1989;84.251-7.

OLITA.

The treatment programme that most comprehensively incorporated all these principles and applied them for a long period was developed in Germany. The patients were certainly concentrated towards the 'difficult' end of the spectrum, as shown by their demographic characteristics. The average age was 43.6 and their alcoholism had lasted for an average of 18.2 years. They had been detoxified as in-patients an average of 7.3 times and were drinking an average of 437.1g of alcohol – the equivalent of well over a bottle of spirits – every day. Their lack of response to all this treatment demonstrated resistance to both the specific and non-specific components of conventional management.[145] Many of them had also received acamprosate without benefit. Naltrexone was not licensed for use in alcoholism for much of the study period but there is no reason to suppose that the results would have been very different. (See Ch. 17)

Yet after two years of treatment, about 75% were staying dry for most of the time, compared with the maximum of 30% expected from comparable studies. Even more importantly, about half of this very unpromising group were *still abstinent after a further seven years* when they were no longer having regular or intensive treatment. In other words, there had been a lasting change for the better in their alcohol-related behaviour. Not surprisingly, this change was accompanied by

---

[145] Krampe H, Stawicki S, Wagner T, Bartels C, Aust C, Rüther E, Poser W, Ehrenreich H. Follow-up of 180 alcoholic patients for up to 7 years after outpatient treatment: impact of alcohol deterrents on outcome. Alc Clin Exp Res. 2006; 30(1):86-95.

favourable changes in their employment status and in the severity of the 'dual diagnosis' psychiatric symptoms that many of them had in addition to their alcoholism.

The main features of OLITA are:

The unusually long duration of the programme (minimum two years);

Frequent short-term contacts with gradual tapering. Initially, this meant 15 minutes daily, "including weekends and holidays", aiming at regular weekly group attendance.

Crisis interventions – which includes the principle that *relapse is an emergency* and that a very brief admission to re-establish abstinence can save a lot of time and money later as well as gaining better long-term outcomes. This, too, was available round-the-clock, weekends and holidays included.[146]

Social re-integration – "assistance in re-arranging a social network which supports an abstinent lifestyle", including, where appropriate, involvement of family members, relationship guidance, help with employment, and financial and legal advice.

Supervised disulfiram (or cyanamide) with appropriate education and advice. Initially - during in-patient

---

[146] The British NHS is unusual among developed nations in the difficulty of obtaining such brief but urgent and useful admissions. It is not difficult in private practice and a bed in a medical ward may be as suitable as a psychiatric one.

detoxification – daily. Then disulfiram 400mg thrice weekly, reducing to twice weekly and once weekly depending on progress, returning to more frequent dosing in the event of lapses or relapses. (A "mini-lapse" was "one single swallow by accident". a "lapse" was drinking for not more than one day. A "relapse" was "recurrence of an addictive drinking pattern with premature termination of treatment". A "malignant relapse" meant refusal of follow-up and loss of contact.)

Regular urine/breath testing for alcohol and other drugs.

Assertive aftercare – "aggressive therapeutic interventions to immediately interrupt...threatening relapses"; spontaneous home visits, telephone calls.

Therapist rotation. The team of 6-7 therapists – psychiatrist, [147] social worker, nurses, students, physician, psychologist[148] – "are equally responsible for all patients".

The importance of continuing disulfiram for long enough to get used to abstinence is shown by the significant increase ($p = <0.001$) in long-term abstinence probability between those who stopped it between 13 and 20 months (50%) and those who took it for >20 months (75%). This is consistent with other research showing that significant changes in self-image took place after about a year and a half of abstinence. Murphy & Hoffman found that alcoholics who had successfully abstained for 18 months had "made a

---

[147] Dr Hannelore Ehrenreich, on of the principal authors.

[148] Dr Henning Krampe, another principal author.

pronounced [cognitive] shift from 'deprived users' to 'determined abstainers'."[149] They were "able to say, 'well, that's how I used to handle these problems, but no longer'."

Of these 180 challenging OLITA patients, *73 did not drink at all*. There were only 8 mini-lapses and 27 lapses. Not surprisingly, the earlier the lapse or relapse, the more likely it was to end unhappily. 115 patients "completed the first year of OLITA with continuous [disulfiram]". The fact that after 13 - 20 months of disulfiram, half the patients achieved lasting abstinence and that after >20 months, 75% of them did so, supports our argument that disulfiram works as an aid to re-education and habit change, although the length of disulfiram treatment was not randomised and the results also reflect patient choice, motivation and preference. The patients who took disulfiram for >20 months actually took it for an average of 976 days. However, once new alcohol-free habits had been established and consolidated (and, just as importantly, become automatic) disulfiram was no longer needed, just as a trainee driver or pilot can eventually drive or fly solo without needing an instructor. Like the OLITA authors, we conclude that the ability of disulfiram to prevent or abort early relapse was a crucially important factor in securing not only an "extraordinary" 50% overall abstinence rate after two years of treatment but also the relative stability of this rate "during the subsequent 7-year observation". Our learning and habituation hypothesis is further supported by the OLITA finding that "the later the first lapse occurs during

---

[149] Murphy S, Hoffman A. 1993. An empirical description of phases of maintenance following treatment for alcohol dependence. J Subst Abuse, 5, 131-143.

long-term abstinence, the more likely it is to [be] cope[d] with". Few clinicians (or patients) would disagree with their contention that "A central therapeutic target, therefore, should be to gain abstinent time".

Two neuroimaging studies also strongly support our argument. Controlled comparisons of expert vs less-expert golfers found significant differences in both the site and the level of brain activity when mentally rehearsing golf swings. The most expert golfers had the lowest levels of activity and fewer areas were involved.[150] The authors suggest that the differences reflect a higher level of automaticity in experts and less interference from the need to decide or think about what to do. "The fact that these differences are apparent before the golfer swings the club suggests that the disparity between the quality of the performance of novice and expert golfers lies at the level of the organization of neural networks during motor planning. In particular, we suggest that extensive practice over a long period of time leads experts to develop a focused and efficient organization of task-related neural networks, whereas novices have difficulty in filtering out irrelevant information".[151] Similarly, in surgical practice, "...a defining trait of experts is that they move more and more problem- solving into an automatic mode".[152]

---

[150] Ross JS, Tkach J, Ruggieri PM, et al. (2003) The mind's eye: functional MR imaging evaluation of golf motor imagery. Am J Neuroradiol 24:1036–44.
[151] Milton J, Solodkin A, Hlustík P, et al. (2007) The mind of expert motor performance is cool and focused. Neuroimage 35:804–13.
[152] Leape L. Cited by Gawande A. (2003) Complications: a surgeon's notes on an imperfect science. 2003; London. Profile. 39.

The only area where we disagree with the conclusions of the OLITA authors is in their contention that the dose of disulfiram does not need to be increased if patients risk drinking without experiencing a DAR and as discussed in Chs. 8 and 9, we are not alone in this view. In support of their contention, they cite the experience of a small (15/180) sub-group of their patients who had medical conditions that were thought to contra-indicate disulfiram and were therefore given – without their knowledge – 'sham' (i.e. placebo) medication. This group had an even higher probability of lasting abstinence (86%) than the 'verum' (i.e. true disulfiram) patients, but for two reasons this is what would be expected. Firstly, among a well-supported group of patients in whom age and/or alcoholism had caused particularly serious physical illness, we would expect poor health to be a factor that independently added to their motivation to abstain, just as some smokers stop smoking after experiencing particularly severe chest or heart problems, or after developing lung cancer.

Secondly, since the risks of the DAR were presumably emphasised and embellished in this group, we would expect the deterrent effect of both real and sham disulfiram to be even greater, with the result that fewer of them would take the risk in the first place. Interestingly, the risk of 'lapses' in this group (as opposed to 'relapses') was similar to the overall rate at around 25%.

If 'lapses' generally meant stopping medication for a day or two but not for long enough to drink much, or at all, that would also be unsurprising. More than half the lapses "occurred within 14 days of the last [disulfiram] intake", so the finding that "experience of [a DAR] after ethanol consumption was rare" is not surprising either. The fact that so many patients were evidently willing to return to the protection provided by disulfiram indicates that they, too, recognised its value and effectiveness. The OLITA authors also note that experiencing a DAR did not make for better results but we would expect and predict that particularly ambivalent patients who were prepared to risk drinking in the hope that they would not experience a DAR (and would therefore be able to continue drinking) would have worse outcomes than less ambivalent patients.

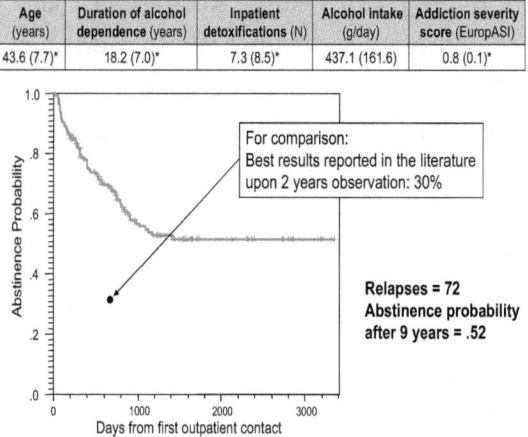

Given such impressive outcomes, it would be churlish to make too much of this point but the experience of the New Zealand study and of Bickel et al, discussed earlier in the book, does suggest that the unprecedentedly positive outcomes of OLITA might have been marginally improved if a few patients who drank without a DAR early in treatment had been offered a higher dose. The evidence suggests that some of them would have accepted and even welcomed the increased deterrent effect at a time when their motivation and belief in their ability to change were still relatively low. If the increased dose meant that they stayed in the programme for long enough to benefit from the other components rather than leaving prematurely, they would probably have added to the "extraordinary" numbers who achieved lasting abstinence.

(More OLITA graphs and tables viewable on www.planetservetus.org)

Chapter 12. A COUNTER-INTUITIVE APPLICATION: using disulfiram in controlled drinking programmes

It is widely assumed that disulfiram can only be appropriate and useful in treatment programmes that have abstinence as their aim. Disulfiram is certainly useful for getting patients to stop drinking but they do not necessarily have to stop for good. Many patients ask whether they will ever be able to drink 'normally' and long-term follow-up research suggests that the correct answer for quite a few of them is a qualified affirmative. In any case, even if advised not to do so, many patients will try. It seems sensible to advise them that if they are thinking of making the experiment, it is better to do so in a planned way so that if it fails, as it often will, there is a rapid-response backup plan

In practice, there are two ways in which disulfiram can be used as part of a controlled drinking programme. One is by using it as a temporary deterrent to drinking in high-risk situations. This is quite commonly suggested in some countries, though patients who have successfully abstained from alcohol for lengthy periods but wish to be able to drink occasionally, often work this out for themselves.[153] In some ways, it is similar to the idea of taking naltrexone intermittently with the aim of limiting drinking to safe levels. However, if naltrexone does not work in this context (and as discussed in Ch. 17, the superiority of naltrexone compared to placebo is not great) then disulfiram is an effective

---

[153] Öjehagen A, Berglund M. To keep the alcoholic in out-patient treatment: a differentiated approach through treatment contracts. Acta Psych Scand 1986;73;68-75

alternative. Patients sometimes discover by experimentation how long it takes for the ALDH-inhibiting effect of disulfiram to wear off, and whether the duration of inhibition is affected by the dose. They then take disulfiram on the same day that they expect to encounter the risky situation or a day or two in advance. While patients who have already developed this level of control and self-control may by that time be able to take disulfiram reliably without supervision, this kind of intermittent use can obviously be incorporated into a supervised programme by arrangement with a spouse or work colleague.

A variant of this approach, noted earlier, is described in a published case report in which the patient, after experimenting unsuccessfully with consistent abstinence, with and without disulfiram, and conventional controlled drinking [154], worked out a programme of supervised disulfiram that was designed to cope with his own particular pattern of drinking. He was a civil servant whose problem drinking occurred only during weekday evenings after work. At weekends he never had a problem and he and his wife could get through a bottle of wine between them at mealtimes without loss of control or problematic behaviour. Eventually, he established a regular pattern of taking 100mg of disulfiram under his wife's supervision every Monday, Tuesday and Wednesday. ALDH inhibition persisted until Friday and by the following day, he could enjoy his normal weekend Shiraz. By the time of publication, he had been

---

[154] Conventional, that is, for most British alcoholism services.

doing this for about 14 years and expected that he would continue with it indefinitely.[155]

A planned treatment programme using somewhat similar principles had been described in a couple of little-known Japanese publications by Mukasa et al using the shorter acting alcohol deterrent calcium cyanamide (still available in some countries).[156,157] The main difference was that instead of adjusting the size and timing of the dose to permit enzymatically-unconstrained controlled drinking only at weekends, the medication was taken every day but with the dose titrated to permit daily drinking up to the point where the reaction with alcohol began to become unpleasant. They called their technique 'Sesshu Ryoho' ('temperance therapy'). In most cases, the drug was taken, and the dosage titrated, in a process of cooperation between the male patients and their wives. However, although the idea is always condemned in Western textbooks, it is or was apparently acceptable for Japanese wives to put an individually tailored dose of cyanamide into the food or drink of uncooperative husbands to at least limit their alcohol intake. It appears that in India, where many drugs are available without prescription, using disulfiram in this way is also not unknown. Since, as previously discussed, about 50% of Japanese men experience partial ALDH inhibition and

---

[155] Brewer C. Using disulfiram to maintain controlled drinking: A case report with a 14-year follow-up. Addict Res 1996;3:231-235
[156] Mukasa H, Ichihara T, Eto A. A new treatment of alcoholism with cyanamide Kurume Med J 1964;11;2,96-101
[157] Mukasa H, Arikawa K. A new double medication method for the treatment of alcoholism using the drug cyanamide. Kurume Med J 1968;15;3,137-43

therefore already get a mild degree of flushing after alcohol[158] that amounts to the effect of an inadequate dose of disulfiram (or cyanamide), it is just about conceivable that they would regard an increase in this flushing to a level that caused serious discomfort as just a natural change in bodily functions, much the same as starting to put on weight after years of slimness or becoming less agile on the tennis court.

I was involved – not as clinician but as an expert witness – in a case where this technique had been successfully used in a world-famous alcoholic – the celebrated jazz musician Stan Getz. The reason that the case can be described here is that it formed an important part of the evidence in his very public divorce case. And also that Stan's widow, Monica, not only agrees that the story can be told but has added some interesting clinical, domestic and historical details.

CASE HISTORY.

I had heard of Stan even before Monica telephoned one day out of the blue - and also about his frequent arrests for drunkenness and heroin abuse, though none of that stopped him from being a great musician or from making a lot of money from his art. I never met Stan himself but I can imagine that he was not the easiest of people to live with.

---

[158] There is a theoretical possibility that regularly raising acetaldehyde levels by drinking while ALDH is inhibited by pharmacological or genetic processes might increase the risk of some cancers, since acetaldehyde is moderately carcinogenic. However, the risk seems to be small, especially when compared to the risks of continuing alcohol abuse and the highest incidence of the cancers thought to be most relevant is not in Japan but in South Asian countries.

Nevertheless, he had been in his second marriage for over twenty years. Monica was an aristocratic Swede, the daughter of a famously anti-Nazi Swedish orthopaedic surgeon and had evidently preserved, along with her beauty, the saintliness necessary to this challenging matrimonial enterprise. On the abundantly documented evidence of Stan's frequent alcoholic binges, with occasional diversions into heroin and cocaine, Monica could have divorced him easily and profitably several times over. She says that she chose not to because they were very much in love and Stan's good periods compensated for his bad ones, even though those often included physical attacks on her but the reasons she hadn't divorced him are not important. The reason for the phone call was that Stan was suing *her* for divorce and his chief complaint involved the technique described above.

Over the years, Monica had become something of an expert on the various types of alcoholism treatment and had even helped with setting up some programmes in her native Sweden. Being an expert in America at that time was fairly easy, because most treatment involved regular attendance at AA groups – and not much else. Things have changed a little since then but only a little. As may easily be imagined, people like Stan Getz don't always find AA groups suited to their individualistic, creative and often rather raucous approach to life. Submerging your identity in that of the group is easier if you don't have much identity to submerge and if you think the group is right. Stan evidently waved two fingers at both notions and continued the familiar cycle of bingeing, drying-out and relapsing.

At some stage, Monica consulted a wise old bird called Ruth Fox. Dr Fox (one of whose disulfiram papers is referenced earlier in the book) was a highly respected US alcoholism specialist in the 1950s and 60s and her name is still commemorated in a prestigious series of lectures organised annually by the American Society of Addiction Medicine. Stan was being impossible again and Monica was almost ready to give up the struggle. She asked if there was anything else – *anything* – that might be tried. Ruth Fox said yes, there was, but it was absolutely a last resort. In the past, some of Stan's doctors had advised him to take disulfiram. (Monica's family knew both Dr Jacobsen and Dr Martensen-Larsen well.) At times, he had taken it regularly and stayed dry for long periods but now, unfortunately, he was refusing it. In this desperate situation, Dr Fox said, there was a case for slipping some into his coffee without telling him. Whether or not it works with alcoholic Japanese husbands, it worked quite well with Stan. Monica slipped him the first dose and when Stan came home later that day, he said that he must have become allergic to alcohol because drinking made him feel ill and he stopped drinking for quite some time. Did he really not suspect the cause of his new 'allergy', or did he suspect it but then decide that this might actually be a way for him to interrupt his alcoholism without losing face? Monica thinks it was probably the latter but who knows and – up to a point – who cares, provided that it stopped him from drinking to excess. Obviously, it only worked while they were still together but that was quite a long period.

Until a few weeks before Monica phoned me, Stan had never mentioned disulfiram even after they split up again but now he was filing for divorce and one of his grounds was that Monica had endangered his life by surreptitiously administering disulfiram.

Monica wanted a disulfiram expert and Ruth Fox herself couldn't help because she had been in a nursing home with Alzheimer's for several years. However, Monica had told her story to a British doctor who happened to be sitting next to her on a plane and he had suggested my name. Stan's lawyers were claiming that disulfiram was a terribly dangerous drug and that slipping it into his tea disqualified Monica from getting a reasonable share of the estate. The fact that Stan had survived several attempts to drink while taking it suggested that it couldn't have been very dangerous in his case and anyway, he had been dangerously near drinking himself to death on several occasions without any help from disulfiram. Monica hoped that I would be able to assist her lawyers.

The Getz home was a former steel magnate's Scottish Baronial palace set in nine acres of very expensive landscape sloping down to the Hudson River, half an hour north of Manhattan by train or, in my case, by Monica's stately white Cadillac. It was very atmospheric and I could see why Monica was reluctant to lose it. The legal battle took place in the courtroom at White Plains, an unremarkable outer suburb that is probably the New York equivalent of Edgware, Ealing or Moonee Ponds. Though I had not previously given evidence in an American court, I felt instantly at home because the whole thing was straight out of any number of Hollywood courtroom dramas. After Monica's lawyer had taken me through my evidence, Stan's attorney rose. To say that he took the stage is not a cliché because he had quite literally brought his stage with him. Courtroom lawyers the world over have a large streak of theatricality and British lawyers are hardly deficient in this respect but in British courts, there are certain procedural and architectural constraints. British barristers don't move about much and they do their stuff from behind a bench or table. As well as the theatrical costumes - the wigs and the gowns - they may have a few theatrical props – large law books or sometimes a small folding bookstand – but they don't stray far from them and they certainly don't pace around or march menacingly up to the dock or the witness box.

Not so in America, where, as every filmgoer knows, they have the run of the space between the public benches, the judge, the accused, other lawyers, the jury and the witness. There, they practise their ancient art, often interestingly close to the even older art of the market trader, with its exaggerated claims and dismissals of doubts, its beguiling mixture of *suggestio falsi* and *suppressio veri*. Even, if defeat seems likely, the resort to bargaining. There they pace, gesture, glare, pause for long periods, blow their noses, clean their spectacles, point their fingers, consult their books and adjust their gowns. These are the lawyerly equivalents of the things that tennis stars do when preparing to serve or receive at Wimbledon, in order to disconcert or distract their opponents. Perhaps younger and more athletic lawyers could try handstands, *entrechats* or *fouettes* as well. Stan's lawyer eschewed these tired old gambits, substituting instead a technique for which not even Hollywood had prepared me. His prop was nothing as simple as a book-rest: it was a whole, almost cathedral-style, lectern. Somebody must have told him at law school that if he carried this lectern into the arena and gradually moved it and himself closer to his victim, it would have a demoralising or even terrifying effect, like the first use of tanks on the Western front in the First World War.

Unfortunately, the attorney was just a shade too small, and the lectern just a shade too large and heavy, for him to carry off this scheme with dignity and without obvious effort. The effect it had on me was not fear but hilarity, especially as most of his questions were based on typically American medical misconceptions about the use and dangers of disulfiram. As an American, he could not understand how someone could be given disulfiram – and perhaps any other medication - without first having a complete battery of blood tests, x-rays and electrocardiograms.

This is not what usually happens in Europe. He was also convinced that if someone taking disulfiram swallowed a small piece of *coq au vin* or splashed some after-shave on his skin, they would have to be rushed to the nearest Emergency Room. The truth is that neither of these minimal exposures to alcohol has any significant pharmacological effect, though patients sometimes get a severe panic attack if they suddenly realise that they have unwittingly swallowed a tiny amount of alcohol and mistakenly think that they are about to get a reaction.

Stan Getz sat impassively through this performance at the back of the court. He won in White Plains but lost his case when it went to appeal.[159] Within a decade, in 1991, he was dead at only 64 from liver cancer, possibly related to viral hepatitis from needle-sharing during his previous heroin habit. He certainly didn't have the ultimate alcoholic's revenge of outliving most of his doctors.

---

[159] Monica put her experience to good use by becoming the founder and President of Coalition for Family Justice, 'a...non-profit service and organization to help children and families resolve family conflicts'.

Chapter 13. DISULFIRAM TREATMENT IN SPECIAL POPULATIONS

We believe that as a general principle, *all* alcoholism treatment should be tailored to the needs of the individual patient. Since there are no specific features of *disulfiram treatment* in women, adolescents or ethnic minorities that are notably different from those of other groups, we do not discuss them.

ALCOHOLIC PHYSICIANS, PILOTS AND OTHER PROFESSIONALS.

Alcoholic physicians differ in several important respects from other alcoholics. First of all, they tend to have a good prognosis and this is partly because they are usually both employable and employed but also because the penalties for relapsing are often both severe and predictable. Depending on the history and severity of the problem, there may be no immediate indication for disulfiram treatment and it can be kept in reserve. However, where a physician has previously come before professional bodies because of alcoholism but has not responded well to treatment, disulfiram is probably indicated and should certainly be considered.

Since doctors understand the mechanism and pharmacology of disulfiram treatment, they may be tempted more than other patients to test out its enzyme-inhibiting ability and therefore this may be one of the situations where there is a case for administering a challenge dose of alcohol to confirm that the dose of disulfiram is adequate. Just as important as disulfiram in this sort of case is monitoring that also takes account of the special ability of doctors to deceive both the treatment team and professional bodies. Supervision of disulfiram can often be done by colleagues but provided the supervisor is acceptable both to the patient and to those bodies, the choice may not be too important. However, physicians and pilots take holidays and go to conferences. Supervision may not be possible on such occasions and the risk of relapse in very ambivalent patients may be high. Some patients, including some doctors, get an understandable but unfortunate satisfaction from trying to beat the system, especially in the early stages of treatment. The full range of monitoring techniques may therefore have to be considered, in part to discourage the patient from even thinking about cheating.

It is particularly important that a full range of blood tests be taken at the first appointment. As well as such standard markers of alcohol abuse as MCV, liver functions, gamma GT and Carbohydrate-Deficient Transferrin, a sample of hair should also be taken – preferably from the scalp but from any other site if necessary. If any of the blood tests show changes typical of alcohol abuse, they should be repeated at weekly or fortnightly intervals after the initial samples and if the patient has abstained during that period, any abnormalities should soon disappear unless serious liver damage has occurred. Further tests for positive markers may be done regularly and/or at random. However, not all patients show abnormalities even if they have been regularly drinking large amounts.

In these cases, testing of hair samples for alcohol metabolites such as ethyl glucuronide[160] will nearly always be positive and if drinking stops completely, a hair sample taken two or three months later should be negative or show very much lower levels, since some hair will be in the resting stage of growth and may not grow at the same rate as the majority of hairs on the sample. Eventually, though, it should become completely negative. If a doctor knows that even occasional drinking will almost certainly be revealed by hair testing, it will probably be easier for him to resist the temptation. Conversely, if the professional bodies have clear evidence from hair tests or blood tests that drinking is continuing, they can take appropriate steps to protect the public by temporarily or permanently suspending the practitioner or by requiring him to practice only in a specialty that does not involve direct risk to patients.

In other respects, treatment is not usually very different from the treatment of patients in similar occupational classes, except that even if the patient seems to be making very good progress, the professional bodies may require treatment and/or monitoring to be continued for a longer period than might be appropriate in less demanding and sensitive occupations. That is certainly true of alcoholic airline pilots.

FAMILY COURTS AND CHILD CARE AND CUSTODY.

Alcohol abuse commonly features in child custody cases and care proceedings, either alone or combined with other drug

---

[160] www.soht.org/images/pdf/2014%20Alcohol%20markers%20revision%2013JUN14%20FINAL.pdf

problems. Encouraging an alcoholic parent or partner to take disulfiram under supervision not only improves the likelihood of sustained abstinence but may also enable judges to feel that the patient is taking the problem seriously. The court may also be reassured that appropriate baseline testing, followed by regular and/or random monitoring has a high likelihood of detecting non-compliance.

PATIENTS FACING TRIAL FOR SERIOUS ALCOHOL-RELATED OFFENCES.

The management of patients taking disulfiram as one condition of a probation order has already been described in Ch. 10. However, where the offence involves serious alcohol-related violence, the courts are understandably reluctant to consider non-custodial sentences. A prison sentence may be unavoidable but may also be changed to probation on appeal. If not, at some stage the prisoner may become eligible for parole. In both cases, if the offender is released on bail pending trial, the pre-sentencing period provides an opportunity not just for preparing a medical report but also for engaging him in treatment. If disulfiram is part of that treatment, as it often should be, that period, typically lasting several months before a Crown Court hearing, enables the physician to document not just continued abstinence, if that has happened, but the likely success of probation-linked treatment if the court is so minded. Good compliance with disulfiram treatment may also persuade a court to defer sentencing and bring the offender back to court from time to time for interim reports. Alternatively, after a few months in prison, the success of pre-trial alcoholism treatment and the fail-safe mechanisms inherent in probation-linked disulfiram may persuade the judges in the Court of Appeal, even if they failed to convince the judges in the Crown Court.

As with the alcoholic physicians and pilots discussed earlier, blood and hair samples should be obtained as soon as possible after the offence. If, as often happens, the defence asks for a medical report while the offender is remanded in prison pending a bail hearing, the visiting physician should take appropriate tubes and phlebotomy needles to collect samples, since blood tests may not have been done, or if done may not have been comprehensive. A hair sample should also be taken and can be tested for other substances as well as alcohol metabolites. The blood and hair samples provide a baseline for future monitoring but if LFTs, for example, are very high but quickly fall with prison-enforced abstinence, they may help to reassure the court that as well as missing a dose of supervised disulfiram, regular testing will quickly detect and thus additionally deter any covert return to heavy drinking.

Particularly if the offender is facing a lengthy sentence, it is worth requesting a CT or MRI brain scan and neuropsychological testing to look for signs of brain damage due both to alcohol and to repeated head injuries from getting into fights. Clear evidence of atrophy or impairment will not (and probably should not) automatically lead to a shorter prison sentence but if there are extenuating circumstances and the court is looking for reasons for lenience, that evidence may be useful. In some cases, it may impress the offender with the need to stop further damage to his brain. As with probation-linked treatment in general, the courts do not need to be persuaded that the offender will not offend again. All they need is to accept that there is a good chance that he will remain sober and stop assaulting the public for at least as long as he would do if they sent him to prison.

ALCOHOLIC METHADONE MAINTENANCE PATIENTS

The incidence of alcoholism among methadone maintenance (MM) patients varies. Many heroin addicts drink little or no alcohol and rarely begin drinking during courses of methadone. However, large surveys show that as many as a third of methadone patients may have significant alcohol problems and not surprisingly, this affects their management and prognosis. Some methadone or buprenorphine programmes have rather punitive attitudes to patients who drink excessively but patients whose alcoholism makes them poor attenders and uncooperative with counselling can try the patience of the most tolerant clinicians. Fortunately, it is usually quite easy to persuade MM patients to begin treatment with disulfiram, provided that taking it is made a condition of continuing in the programme, or of continued privileges such as take-home methadone. Nearly all methadone patients with alcohol problems regard their methadone as more important and irreplaceable than their alcohol and if required to take disulfiram, they will not usually argue too much. If there is a choice of maintenance programmes in their area and they threaten to take their custom to a more forgiving clinic, that at least solves the problem for you and your colleagues, even if not for the patient. In practice, as shown in the report by Bickel et al, offering alcoholic MM patients privileges, or continuing them, in exchange for compliance with disulfiram, is a very powerful bargaining chip if the alternative involves transfer to a clinic that may not insist on disulfiram but will insist on indefinite daily pick up. Including Sundays.

As discussed in the dosage section, Bickel et al also showed that if patients taking methadone-linked disulfiram continued to drink on standard doses, progressively increasing the disulfiram dose eventually achieved and maintained abstinence from alcohol. Thus, even with difficult patients, attention to small but important details of treatment means that disulfiram will nearly always 'do what it says on the can', provided the dose is adequate. A few other studies have also combined methadone and disulfiram in this way with consistently beneficial effects. As yet, no study involving disulfiram and buprenorphine (or slow release oral morphine) has been published but the principles are identical and there is no reason to suppose that the results would be any different.

ALCOHOLIC COCAINE ABUSERS

Some cocaine-abusing patients regularly use alcohol either to 'come down' from a cocaine high, or as a regular addition, and sometimes a regular precursor, to their use of cocaine. Some patients report that they would use less or no cocaine if they did not drink at the same time, because alcohol either reduces some of the unpleasant effects of cocaine or reduces their resistance to the temptation to use it. In such cases, disulfiram can have obvious and useful effects in either reducing cocaine use or enabling the patient to abstain completely. As with abstinence from alcohol, abstinence from cocaine will almost certainly reinforce the specific and non-specific effects of whatever psychological or psychosocial treatment may also be indicated.

Early reports indicated that disulfiram might also be helpful in cocaine abuse even in patients who were not drinking heavily. The results of these studies have not been consistently replicated and it is not clear what the relevant mechanisms might be, or the optimum dosage and length of treatment. Interference with dopamine metabolism is a possible candidate.

DETOXIFIED FORMER HEROIN OR METHADONE USERS WHO START OR RESUME ALCOHOL ABUSE.

Although many opiate-dependent patients do not have alcohol problems while they are using heroin, methadone, or buprenorphine, it is not at all uncommon for patients to start drinking heavily after successful withdrawal from opiates. In some cases, this represents the return of previous alcoholism that has been in abeyance (or less of a problem) while the patient was opiate dependent. In others, it represents an understandable response by the patient to the discomforts and anxieties of the first month or two after opiate withdrawal and the worrying novelty of living in an unintoxicated state. Naturally, some patients respond to this by quickly relapsing to opiates rather than using alcohol but in patients who remain opiate free by their own efforts or, increasingly, with the assistance and protection of depot or implanted preparations of naltrexone, significant and persistent alcohol abuse poses an obvious threat to their current well-being and future recovery.

The relative ineffectiveness of naltrexone in alcohol abuse compared with disulfiram is discussed in Ch. 17. In no clinical situation is this ineffectiveness more apparent than when patients with adequate and consistent blood levels from oral or depot naltrexone start drinking heavily after opiate withdrawal. Only one study, in 132 patients, seems to have examined this but the results are clear. "We found a significant increase of the amount of alcohol consumed, that was higher in the patients who had shown alcohol abuse before opiate dependence."[161]

Heavy drinking immediately after opiate withdrawal is quite often a short-lived problem that abates without treatment during the first month, when most of the residual discomforts of withdrawal have usually disappeared. If it continues, or if it is sufficiently severe straight after withdrawal to be an obvious problem, then disulfiram can be added to naltrexone treatment if a suitable supervisor can be found. In many cases, patients at this stage of treatment after opiate withdrawal will be in some sort of regular treatment or counselling programme and disulfiram can easily be supervised by treatment staff if there are no ideological

---

[161] Ochoa Mangado E, Arias Horcajadas F. Consumo de alcohol en dependientes de opiáceos en tratamiento con naltrexona. Actas Esp Psiquiatr 2000;28:239-249.

objections. There are no known adverse interactions between the two drugs.

A WORD ABOUT NALTREXONE AND LIVER DISEASE.

Some clinicians are anxious about using naltrexone or disulfiram in a group of patients with a high incidence of chronic hepatitis B or C, some of whom have persistent abnormalities of liver function tests. The safety of disulfiram in this situation is discussed in the next chapter. Fortunately, despite persistent claims to the contrary, naltrexone is also safe in patients suffering from even life-threatening liver diseases. The most important and impressive evidence for its lack of hepatotoxicity comes not from studies of liver functions in patients with chronic hepatitis but from studies of naltrexone used in a completely different context. Just as disulfiram has useful chelating, anti-parasitic, anti-cancer and anti-glaucoma effects (see Appendix 1), naltrexone also has some unsuspected uses.

One of these is the relief of otherwise intractable itching in patients with severe jaundice due to severe liver disease.[162] It has proved to be both effective for many patients[163] and free of significant side-effects, despite daily doses of more than

---

[162] Terg R, Coronel E, Sorda J, Munoz AE, Findor J. Efficacy and safety of oral naltrexone treatment for pruritus of cholestasis: a crossover, double blind, placebo controlled study. J Hepatol 2002. 37(6): 717-722.
[163] Siemens W1, Xander C, Meerpohl JJ, Antes G, Becker G. Drug treatments for pruritus in adult palliative care. Dtsch Arztebl Int. 2014 Dec 12;111(50):863-70. doi: 10.3238/arztebl.2014.0863.

50mg and assorted liver diseases of such severity that in several cases, liver transplantation was being urgently considered. Since naltrexone is safe even in these life-threatening hepatic situations, clinicians need not be very worried about using it in patients with chronic hepatitis that in many cases is not causing any symptoms of liver disease. Even in acute viral hepatitis, it seems to be very safe.[164] If LFT monitoring is thought to be needed, it should be occasional rather than intensive.

---

[164] Brewer C, Wong V-S. Naltrexone: a case report of lack of hepatotoxicity in acute viral hepatitis, with a review of the literature. Addiction Biol 2004; 9: 81-7.

Chapter 14. 'SAFER THAN ASPIRIN': the side-effects of disulfiram

Chapter 8 records the views of several distinguished alcoholism clinicians about some important aspects of disulfiram treatment and their differing attitudes to the balance of risks and benefits may help to put concerns about the safety of disulfiram in perspective. Its supposedly high level of side-effects or Adverse Effects (AEs) is certainly cited by some clinicians (and occasionally by patients) as reasons for reluctance or refusal to use disulfiram. These divide neatly into two categories: its AEs in patients who are successfully deterred from drinking by compliance with regular disulfiram intake; and the consequences of the reaction with alcohol (the Disulfiram-Alcohol Reaction – DAR) if they have not been sufficiently deterred to risk drinking.

Disulfiram does not have a particularly high incidence of AEs when compared with other drugs. As noted in the Copenhagen symposium, it was classed as 'intermediate' in a Danish governmental review[165] and most AEs of disulfiram are both minor and short-lived, such as tiredness and (usually) mild headache. We believe Gitlow was correct in his view that disulfiram is "safer than aspirin".[166] Many other

---

[165] Poulson EH, Loft S, Andersen JR, Andersen M. Disulfiram therapy – adverse drug reactions and interactions. Acta Psychiat Scandinav 1992;86:59-66.
[166] Gitlow SE. Antabuse. In Gitlow SE, Peyser HS Alcoholism: a practical treatment guide. New York, Grune and Stratton, 1980; 273. Note for the unmedical: Aspirin can cause rare and often fatal disorders

drugs may also cause AEs at the start of treatment that soon disappear or become less apparent as the body adapts. Taking disulfiram at night may solve the problem of tiredness and in the early stages of treatment it may even improve sleep if it is disturbed by persistent alcohol withdrawal symptoms. A garlic-like odour on the breath is sometimes noticed by others but is rarely a problem. During the first two or three decades of disulfiram treatment, national pharmacopoeias commonly suggested that if drugs like anticonvulsants or antihistamines (or, by implication, disulfiram) caused troublesome daytime tiredness, a stimulant such as dexamphetamine or methylphenidate could be added to offset it. That was very much frowned on by the 1990s but now that such drugs are being prescribed so freely to children, adolescents and adults with real or alleged ADHD, the very occasional sleepy disulfiram patient can surely be helped to stay awake during the day without much risk to the health of the nation. In any case, since disulfiram consumption should always be supervised, the supervisor can and should look after any stimulants as well and dispense them in small installments.

---

such as Reye's Disease but the main risks come from direct irritation of the stomach causing ulcers and perforation; and from its anticoagulant properties which mean that any cause of external or internal bleeding may have much more serious consequences, including death. Alcoholics with gastritis and gastric ulcers, or portal hypertension and oesophageal varices, are probably much more at risk of dying from aspirin-enhanced bleeding than from treatment with disulfiram.

SKIN AND THE NICKEL FACTOR.

Disulfiram rarely causes rashes. When it does, they usually appear in areas that have previously been in contact with nickel-containing rings and other adornments. This is because disulfiram powerfully chelates (i.e. binds with) nickel and several other metallic ions including copper, cobalt and lead. It can therefore drag out tiny quantities of nickel that have been lurking in adjacent skin and subcutaneous tissues, or more generally, and briefly enable it to cause toxic or allergic reactions. Nickel is a common cause of rashes and disulfiram is one of the drugs used by dermatologists to remove residual nickel if it is causing chronic dermatitis. If rashes appear in areas suggestive of present or former nickel contact, disulfiram should not routinely be discontinued but corticosteroid creams should be applied to the inflamed area. Within a week or two, the chelated nickel will usually be excreted and the rash will disappear. Typical generalized drug rashes are very rarely seen. If they are severe and persist despite corticosteroids, it may be impossible to continue disulfiram but I have never seen such a case.

NEUROLOGICAL ADVERSE EFFECTS.

Classic peripheral neuropathy is an uncommon but well-recognised AE of disulfiram, as it is of many other commonly prescribed drugs. It may be related to hydrogen sulphide (H_2S) which is a metabolite of disulfiram and probably accounts for the occasional garlic-like odour as well. Neuropathy is dose-related[167] and most cases involve doses of more than 250mg/day.[168] Some patients only developed neuropathy when the dose was increased. In one report, it appeared when the dose was changed, for what was described as 'no particular reason', from 500mg to 1000mg/day.[169] As discussed in the section on dosage in Ch. 9, most patients do not need doses of more than about 200mg/day and are thus unlikely to experience neuropathy.

Another common feature of reported cases involving alcoholism treatment is that several weeks passed between the onset of typical neuropathic symptoms and the diagnosis of neuropathy. Sometimes, this reflected an apparent failure to see the patient for early review but in others, obvious symptoms seem to have been unnoticed or ignored at consultations. In one of my own cases, the private GP who referred the patient insisted – for what seemed to be primarily financial reasons – on seeing the patient weekly himself for the month after her first consultation, instead of letting me do it. At her first follow-up visit with me a month later, it was obvious from the difficulty with which she mounted the stairs to my consulting-room that something was badly wrong but the GP had not noticed her obvious neuropathy. She later successfully sued the GP for missing the diagnosis. In

---

[167] Frisoni GB, Di Monda V. Disulfiram neuropathy: a review (1971-1988) and report of a case. Alcohol Alcohol. 1989;24(5):429-37.
[168] Dano P, Tammam D, Brosset C, Bregigeon M. [Peripheral neuropathies caused by disulfiram]. Rev Neurol (Paris). 1996 Apr;152(4):294-5.
[169] Dandelot J-B, Dupuis M. L'Antabuse: ange ou demon? [review of disulfiram neuropathy] *Le* Concours Medical 1979: 101; 7666-73.

another particularly severe reported case, [170] symptoms appeared one month after disulfiram was started at the needlessly high dose of 500mg/day. The classic clinical picture of severe generalized neuropathy "progressed over six weeks with speech impairment, difficulty in swallowing liquids and inability to walk" with cranial nerve involvement before somebody recognized it, by which time urgent admission was needed. Only then was disulfiram stopped. Fortunately, the patient made a partial recovery, though six months later, he still needed crutches to get about. The story arguably says more about the prescribing clinician or the follow-up arrangements than about disulfiram.

The simplest way to avoid disulfiram neuropathy is to tell patients that it can sometimes occur and what symptoms should make them suspect it. If disulfiram is stopped at the first sign of trouble, neuropathy – which may very rarely involve the optic nerve - always disappears quickly. If stopping disulfiram makes managing the alcohol problem difficult, continuing at a smaller dosage with careful monitoring may solve the problem. At one time, the alternative alcohol-sensitising drug cyanamide could be substituted but it is no longer easily available in most countries.

---

[170] Santos T, Martins Campos A, Morais H. Sensory-motor axonal polyneuropathy involving cranial nerves: An uncommon manifestation of disulfiram toxicity. Clin Neurol Neurosurg. 2017 Jan;152:12-15. doi: 10.1016/j.clineuro.2016.11.005. Epub 2016 Nov 10.

DISULFIRAM AND THE LIVER.

Disulfiram's only life-threatening AE is a hepatitis that can be so severe and rapid in onset that it attracts the adjective 'fulminating'.[171] The first point to make is that in some four decades of disulfiram prescribing, I never came across a single case – or heard about one from colleagues. Large-scale surveys from national reporting agencies confirm both that it can be lethal and that it is rare – one death in 25,000 patient treatment years.[172] However, death from this cause is almost always avoidable. Like neuropathy, hepatitis usually appears in the first 1 – 3 months of treatment and as with neuropathy, a feature of several reported cases is the generally inexcusable delay between the first signs of hepatitis and the discontinuation of disulfiram after diagnosis.

As with neuropathy, the first step in avoiding the development of severe hepatitis is to warn and educate patients and their GPs appropriately and routinely. Easy reporting access to the prescriber or to properly-informed members of the treatment team is important but in these days of text-messages and emails, that should not be difficult even if patients do not have direct telephone access (which should be routine in private practice at least). Immediate withdrawal of disulfiram at the first sign of trouble seems to be always followed by rapid recovery. Although it probably would not be thought wise in today's more litigious atmosphere, in

---

[171] From the Latin *fulmen* – a lightning flash.
[172] Poulson EH, Loft S, Andersen JR, Andersen M. Disulfiram therapy – adverse drug reactions and interactions. Acta Psychiat Scand 1992;86:59-66.

some early case reports, patients were challenged with disulfiram after recovery to confirm that it was disulfiram that caused the hepatitis rather than some other cause – e.g. a virus, or a different drug. Even when the challenge duly caused further symptoms and abnormalities in liver function tests (LFTs) no patient suffered lasting harm. As Chick reminds us, severe hepatitis from any cause always makes patients feel unwell.[173] If that alone does not lead them to contact the prescriber or the treatment team, the appearance of classic dark urine or yellow eyeballs certainly should, yet these obvious signs were either not reported (because patients were not warned about them) or the mainly psychiatric physicians who were responsible for the medical aspects of follow-up did not ask about them, or notice them.

It should go without saying that if the follow-up is done by personnel without a medical or nursing background, they should be trained to look for and ask about the very obvious and classic signs and symptoms, as well as about neuropathic ones. Such familiarity with the side effects of common drugs would usually be routine among the non-medical counselling staff in family-planning clinics.[174] Some clinicians advise routine fortnightly and then monthly LFTs in the first few months of disulfiram treatment but patient education and easy access to the prescriber may be more effective as well as less disruptive.

---

[173] Chick J. Safety issues concerning the use of disulfiram in treating alcohol dependence. Drug Safety. 1999;20;427-35.
[174] Brewer C. Editorial (bilingual): Harm-reduction for unwanted pregnancies and unwanted addictions: an instructive analogy. Adicciones, 2008;20(1):5-13

These sagas of missed diagnosis by psychiatrists and generalists make a depressing and shameful contrast with the way in which dermatologists recognize and manage disulfiram hepatitis. As mentioned earlier, dermatologists sometimes use disulfiram to remove nickel from the body in cases of chronic nickel dermatitis. It is a curious but very significant feature of disulfiram treatment for dermatitis rather than alcoholism that far from being very rare, the incidence of raised LFTs was around 20% with frank hepatitis developing in around 10%.[175] The same authors specifically note "the sharp contrast to the few reported side effects when alcoholic patients are treated with disulfiram" and the fact that neither hepatotoxicity nor hepatitis were dose-related.

However, since dermatologists are 'proper' physicians and have no residual Freudian hangups about actually examining their patients, if hepatitis occurs, they tend to notice it. That may explain why no deaths have been reported from disulfiram hepatitis in a dermatological setting. It may also explain another curious feature of disulfiram hepatitis in alcoholism, which is that although male alcoholics commonly outnumber females by anything from 5:1 to 2:1 (the difference is getting smaller as women increasingly drink like men) most reported case series of disulfiram hepatitis in alcoholism have equal or greater numbers of female patients.

---

[175] Kaaber K, Menne T, Veien N, Baadsgaard O. Some adverse effects of fisulfiram in the treatment of nickel-allergic patients. Dermatosen Beruf Umwelt 1987;38;209-11

This strongly suggests that disulfiram hepatitis is not simply due to an inherent hepatotoxicity of disulfiram but to some additional factor that is commoner in women than in men and the obvious candidate is nickel, since women are more likely than men to wear nickel-containing jewellery and to become nickel-sensitive.

Kaabe et al pointed out in 1987 that, "10% of the adult female [Danish] population is sensitized to nickel" and changes in both prosperity and fashion have increased that figure in both sexes. A recent Danish survey[176] upped it to 17% in women and 3% in men and noted that as well as traditional sources such as jewellery, coins and fasteners, nickel in "dental restorations, mobile phones, and leather" contributed to the problem. Therefore, as well as routinely warning and educating patients, it is worth asking them specifically about previous nickel sensitivity when starting disulfiram and urging them to be extra-vigilant if they have ever experienced it.[177] A unique and remarkable case report of severe fulminant hepatitis due to an unsuspected disulfiram implant is discussed in Ch. 18.

Clinicians should also be aware that worrying fluctuations in LFTs may occasionally be due to unremarkable social or gastronomic activities that have nothing to do with either medication or illness. The misleading sensitivity of liver

---

[176] Thyssen JP, Menné T. Metal allergy--a review on exposures, penetration, genetics, prevalence, and clinical implications. Chem Res Toxicol. 2010 Feb 15;23(2):309-18. doi: 10.1021/tx9002726.
[177] Brewer C. Hardt F. Preventing disulfiram hepatitis in alcohol abusers: inappropriate guidelines and the significance of nickel allergy. Addiction Biol 1999;4:303-308

function tests to a number of ordinary environmental toxins was shown in a case report of a patient receiving the opiate antagonist nalmefene. During an experimental study, she developed significant but transient LFT abnormalities, which disappeared spontaneously despite the continuation of nalmefene. They were subsequently thought most likely to have been a response to chillies in Oriental food[178] and it is clear that other incidental and non-pharmacological factors can cause transient LFT abnormalities. For example, Mitchell et al noted a short-lived increase in AST in one of their patients two days after she had taken part in a marathon.[179]

USING DISULFIRAM IN PATIENTS WITH CIRRHOSIS OR ALCOHOLIC HEPATITIS.

Far from being dangerous, prescribing disulfiram for alcoholic patients with seriously disturbed liver functions or frank cirrhosis is regarded by many Danish physicians as both routine and life-saving.[180] In such cases, LFTs will be closely monitored anyway and in the very unlikely event of disulfiram causing a sustained and alarming increase in liver enzymes, or other abnormalities, a decision can be made about continuing treatment. The main problem with using disulfiram in patients with cirrhosis is that in some cases, as mentioned earlier, the biotransformation of disulfiram to its active metabolite may not take place efficiently. Higher

---

[178] Salvato FR, Mason B. Changes in transaminases over the course of a twelve-week, double blind nalmefene trial in a 38-year old female subject. Alcohol Clin Exp Res 1994;18:1187-9

[179] Mitchell JE, Morley JE, Levine AS, Hatsukami D, Gannon M, Pfohl D. High-dose naltrexone therapy and dietary counselling for obesity. Biol Psychiatry 1987;22:35 – 42.

[180] Hardt F. Personal communication.

doses may be needed and in a very few cases, a DAR may not occur. However, like other disulfiram patients, most cirrhotic patients taking disulfiram will not drink either at all or after experiencing a single DAR. Since continuing to drink despite cirrhosis means a high risk of death, the very much smaller risks of trying to treat the cause with disulfiram are negligible in comparison. Kulig et al support this position, arguing that "the risk of disulfiram liver injury appears much lower than that from alcohol" and that "Disulfiram therapy may allow prolonged abstinence leading to successful antiviral therapy for [Hepatitis C], and time to begin behavioral treatments that facilitate long-term abstinence".[181]

CEREBRAL EFFECTS

Large-scale studies have shown that disulfiram is safe to use even in patients with active psychiatric illness and even at the most severe, psychotic end of the spectrum, though good communication with the psychiatric team is obviously important if the alcoholism is being treated separately.[182] However, a very few reports have occurred of confusional states associated with disulfiram. It may be significant that most of these come from India and they may indicate some localized genetic hypersensitivity. One possible mechanism for cerebral effects is the same chelating ability that can cause acute and short-lived exacerbations of nickel

---

[181] Kulig KC, Beresford T. Hepatitis C in Alcohol Dependence: Drinking versus Disulfiram J Addict Dis 2005. 24 (2) 77-89
[182] Larson E, Olincy A, Rummans TA, Morse RM. Disulfiram treatment of patients with both alcohol dependence and other psychiatric disorders: A review. Alc Clin Exp Res 1992;16:125-130.

dermatitis, and provoke hepatitis [183]. As with nickel, disulfiram chelates lead by forming lipid-soluble complexes, which can readily cross the blood-brain barrier. If the body contains small amounts of environmental lead, a short-lived surge in lead levels could adversely affect brain function.[184] Perhaps sub-clinical lead poisoning from lead-containing paint or plumbing is a factor in India. In a report from Japan, confusion developed gradually in the first month of treatment and inadequate follow-up or family and patient education may have delayed the diagnosis. There were EEG abnormalities which resolved, as did the confusion, when disulfiram was discontinued.[185]

Another possible explanation is that if disulfiram is started in physically dependent patients who have only been alcohol free for three or four days, confusional states or organic psychoses could represent a late or atypical manifestation of alcohol withdrawal delirium. I have seen two patients with confusion which settled quickly and have heard about another case in a patient treated elsewhere who had no delirium during several weeks of disulfiram treatment under my care. This patient also had epilepsy that was not always well controlled and could have been a cause of confusion in itself. In one unusual case, a young woman who was taking

---

[183] Zala D, Schmid M, Buhler H. Fulminante hepatitis durch disulfiram. Deutsche Med Wochenschr 1993;118;1355-60
[184] Miller L. Disulfiram-induced lead intoxication. Am J Psychiat 1993;150;7, 1130
[185] Iwashige T, Shibasaki M. [Disulfiram-induced delirium: a case report].
[Article in Japanese] Nihon Arukoru Yakubutsu Igakkai Zasshi. 2006 Dec;41(6):535-40.

amphetamines for ADHD developed a short-lived psychosis when disulfiram was added to her medication.[186] It resolved quickly after both drugs were discontinued. The authors discuss possible mechanisms, including disulfiram's ability to inhibit cerebral dopamine β-hydroxylase but if that was the cause, it is clearly one that affects very few patients.

CARDIOVASCULAR SYSTEM

Textbooks often advise that disulfiram should not be given to patients aged more than 60 or suffering from significant cardiac disease. While caution should certainly be exercised, patients in this category who continue drinking heavily despite other forms of treatment are quite likely to be at greater risk from the alcohol than they would be from the disulfiram, especially since most will probably not risk drinking on it. My oldest disulfiram patient was in his 80s and after he stopped drinking, he began an affair which, from his enthusiastic descriptions, might of itself have caused some cardiac problems. As always, the risks of treatment need to be balanced against the risks of the disorder – a point recognized even by cautious commentators.

PREGNANCY

All drugs should be avoided if possible in pregnancy and

---

[186] Spiegel DR, McCroskey A, Puaa K, Meeker G, Hartman L, Hudson J, Hung YC. A Case of Disulfiram-Induced Psychosis in a Previously Asymptomatic Patient Maintained on Mixed Amphetamine Salts: A Review of the Literature and Possible Pathophysiological Explanations. Clin Neuropharmacol. 2016 Sep-Oct;39(5):272-5. doi: 10.1097/WNF.0000000000000166.

disulfiram is no exception. It is not certain that disulfiram has significant teratogenic effects but it is certain that heavy alcohol consumption does. Fortunately, I have never been faced with the need to consider the use of disulfiram in pregnancy. If it is to be used at all, it should clearly be a last resort and it might be ethically easier to invoke compulsory powers of detention and enforced abstinence to protect the unborn child against foetal alcohol syndrome.

DRUG INTERACTIONS

Disulfiram has few significant interactions with drugs that are likely to be co-prescribed for most alcoholic patients. It may slow the metabolism of some drugs, including anticonvulsants and warfarin, and doses may need to be adjusted accordingly, but apart from drug formulations that include ethyl or other alcohols, the risk of severe interactions seems to be restricted to metronidazole. Some authors are concerned on theoretical grounds about possible interactions with antidepressants but they seem unfounded. As argued earlier, there are very few reasons for initiating antidepressants in the first two or three months after starting disulfiram until consistent abstinence makes an accurate assessment possible but where a patient is already taking antidepressants, there is no need to discontinue them. In the study by Larson et al referenced earlier, the conclusion was that "At the usual dosage, about 250mg/day, disulfiram does not appear to increase significantly the risk of psychiatric complications or of psychiatric drug interactions. Therefore, it can be considered a treatment option for patients with alcohol dependence and other psychiatric disorders." There is a case report in which disulfiram was supervised together with the MAOI-inhibitor tranylcypromine as a last-resort in a patient with both alcohol and cocaine abuse.[187]

THE DISULFIRAM-ALCOHOL REACTION (DAR).

As earlier noted, in the early days of disulfiram treatment, it was common both to give large doses – up to 3000mg/day – and to make patients drink a relatively large amount of alcohol so that they would experience a severe DAR. A few deaths occurred following these alcohol 'challenges'. Since severe alcoholics often have disease or impairment of several organs, including the heart, and since many of them were – and still are – heavy smokers, it is not surprising that some of them experienced life-threatening cardiac reactions. In one fatal case reported as late as the early 1980s in a Belfast newspaper (but not in the medical literature), a patient who had already had a noticeable and unpleasant reaction to a test dose of alcohol was urged by his physician to drink a further dose, following which he quickly collapsed and died. At post-mortem, severe coronary disease was found. Most physicians who use disulfiram seem to think that there is never any need to give a test dose. I think that 'never' is too strong a term and at the end of this chapter, I explain why I believe that it is still occasionally necessary and how to carry it out safely when it is needed.

Most patients who take disulfiram as directed will not risk drinking. If they manage, with the intention of relapsing, to stop disulfiram for long enough to exceed what they believe

---

[187] Brewer C. Treatment of cocaine abuse with monoamine oxidase inhibitors: a case report. Brit J Psychiat 1993;163: 815-6.

to be its duration of effect, they may get an unpleasant surprise if they drink alcohol after three or four days. Occasionally, they will get the same surprise if they wait as long as a week or more. Other patients may drink on the same day that they receive their regular dose in the hope that they will somehow escape the DAR or find it only mildly unpleasant – a point discussed in the section on dosage.

These patients may experience a severe and very unpleasant reaction. The severity depends on the amount of alcohol consumed, the degree of ALDH impairment and other individual factors such the as the reaction of the cardiovascular system to falling or rising blood-pressure and the patient's tendency to vomit or have headaches. The rate at which alcohol, in the first stage of its metabolism, is converted to acetaldehyde by the enzyme alcohol dehydrogenase may also be important and like most of the other factors, may largely be genetically determined.

Although I have some possibly unique colour photographs of patients experiencing a mild DAR in the course of an alcohol challenge, including them in the book would have greatly increased publishing costs and we have therefore made them available on the website instead. As they reveal, the most obvious manifestation of a mild DAR is flushing of the face and chest, usually associated with a fall in blood pressure and a rise in pulse-rate.

The patient shown in Plates 1 and 2 had at one time suffered a perforated gastric ulcer, probably related to his drinking, and the flushing is also noticeable in the area of his mid-line laparotomy scar, as well as in the chest. Although not shown in the picture, it was equally noticeable in the scar on his arm from an old compound fracture that had also been caused by his drinking. Although he had already had a moderate reaction (Plate 1) to the small dose of alcohol that had been administered (12.5ml of 40^0 brandy - about half a unit of alcohol) he said that he was not impressed and requested a bigger dose.

Since he was in a medical hospital, rather than a psychiatric one, with good resuscitation facilities, this was given. Plate 2 shows not only much more widespread flushing but also a stain on his pillow from vomiting. His blood pressure fell slightly but there was no need to call the crash team or administer any other medication or even put him into the head-down position. Not surprisingly, he didn't risk drinking on disulfiram again, though he did try some of the standard tricks to evade it.

No patient of mine died or suffered serious or lasting consequences from drinking while taking disulfiram. There are very few reports of deaths in the literature or in national statistics in the last few decades.[188] However, it should always be impressed on patients that death from the DAR is possible and common sense suggests that emphasizing the risks may help to increase the deterrent effect. Reviewing prescribers' attitudes to disulfiram, a South African pharmacologist criticises their tendency to exaggerate the real risk of a fatal DAR as emphasizing external rather than

---

[188] Chick J. Safety issues concerning the use of disulfiram in treating alcohol dependence. Drug Safety. 1999;20;427-35.

internal motivation and locus of control[189] but at the start of disulfiram treatment, control of drinking is usually the overriding issue, not its precise location within the patient's psychological world. That can be discussed at leisure - and if necessary adjusted - after the dust has settled. Patients – especially depressed patients - should also be told that if they feel tempted to commit suicide by drinking on top of disulfiram, it is likely both to fail and to be a very unpleasant experience. Suicidal overdoses of disulfiram itself are uncommon. This may be because it has no general reputation as an effective drug for this purpose. Lasting damage to deep brain structures has sometimes been reported following disulfiram overdose although patients usually make a reasonable recovery[190] and death appears to be unknown or very rare.

There is usually no need to treat the DAR. If it seems to be nearing life-threatening severity, the production of further acetaldehyde can be completely inhibited by an intravenous infusion of 4-methylpyrrazole. Acetaldehyde that is already present in the blood should then be excreted fairly rapidly via the lung and kidney (it is volatile at body temperature) as well as being metabolised by residual ALDH activity, leading to the gradual disappearance of DAR symptoms, which can meanwhile be managed with ordinary supportive measures if necessary. The antidote is fortunately not easily

---

[189] van Zyl P. Doctors' views of disulfiram and their response to relapse in alcohol-dependent patients, Free State, 2009. Afr J Prim Health Care Fam Med. 2016 Jun 17;8(1):1-7
[190] Lemoyne S, Raemaekers J, Daems J, Heytens L. Delayed and prolonged coma after acute disulfiram overdose. Acta Neurol Belg. 2009 Sep;109(3):231-4.

available to the general public and also very expensive. If it were to become available in an orally active form, it might be used by extremely ambivalent and sophisticated patients as an additional technique for evading or sabotaging treatment but it could presumably be easily detected, if it were suspected, with a blood or urine test. One drug company has proposed to market something similar to make it possible for the many people who experience the Oriental flush to drink alcohol without discomfort.

I naturally (if selfishly and undemocratically) hope that they will not do so. Fortunately, as well as its efficacy, its safety in what would often presumably be lifelong use would take many years to establish. Some patients have read that drugs such as vitamin C or antihistamines can prevent the DAR but none of them seems to have more than modest effects in practice, if that.[191]

Patients often believe that they will immediately vomit if they drink alcohol. If they make the experiment and don't vomit, many will stop when they experience flushing and dizziness. Others may continue until a more severe reaction sets in a few minutes later.

---

[191] Stowell A, Johnsen J, Ripel A, Mørland J. Diphenhydramine and the calcium carbimide-ethanol reaction: a placebo-controlled clinical study. Clin Pharmacol Ther. 1986 May;39(5):521-5.

ADMINISTERING A CHALLENGE DOSE OF ALCOHOL.

There are still a very few occasions when, in my opinion, it is both justifiable and necessary to do an alcohol challenge. One of them is when a patient with a history of many previous unsuccessful treatment episodes without disulfiram has got into one of those 'Five D's' situations where he is very likely to lose his job, his family, his life, his home or his liberty if his alcoholism is not very quickly brought under control. In such situations, an early relapse may make everybody involved in treatment, or associated with the patient finally lose hope.

If his wife leaves him, the courts imprison him, his employer fires him, or his liver incapacitates him, that may turn a difficult situation into a catastrophic and untreatable one. Conversely, even securing a few months of abstinence for the first time may introduce a little optimism. If a patient in this situation tests out the DAR by drinking and finds that the reaction does not deter him, that can be a disaster even if a subsequent dose increase restores sobriety.

The object of the challenge dose is not to make patients feel ill. It is simply to demonstrate to them that even a modest amount of alcohol will produce a modest reaction and that if they drink more than a small amount the reaction will be proportionately more severe. As discussed in the section on dosage, there is no need for the patient to have taken disulfiram for several days at more than the normal daily dosage before its effects begin.

Enzyme inhibition appears to reach the peak level for the dose in question within 24 hours[192] - possibly much sooner[193] - and the challenge dose can be administered any time after that. On an empty stomach, the patient swallows half a unit of undiluted brandy or whisky – i.e. about 12.5ml - or its equivalent. If that is enough to cause a reaction, signs will appear within 15 to 20 minutes. If they do not appear, a whole unit should be given. By that time, the half unit should have been largely metabolised by the body. If there is no reaction after a whole unit, the dose of disulfiram should be increased and the test repeated within a day or two.

Recall that a significant minority of patients get little or no reaction on doses of 200mg even if they do drink large amounts. An alternative approach to establishing the existence of ALDH inhibition is to apply an alcohol-soaked swab to the skin of the forearm. According to a Japanese report using cyanamide, this will produce local flushing of the skin if ALDH inhibition exists but without any systemic effects.[194] The dose needed to produce localised flushing ranged from 30mg to 150mg (the usual cyanamide dose is 50mg). This presumably indicates that with cyanamide as

---

[192] Hart BW, Yourick JJ, Faiman MD. S-methyl-N,N-diethylthiolcarbamate: a disulfiram metabolite and potent rat liver mitochondrial low Km aldehyde dehydrogenase inhibitor. Alcohol. 1990 Mar-Apr;7(2):165-9.

[193] Anecdotally too, enzyme inhibition begins very quickly. One of my patients who had a brief lapse rashly decided to take disulfiram to terminate her drinking. She reported that within 30 minutes, she was violently sick.

[194] Yamauchi M, Kimura T, Takeda K, Sakamoto K, Ohata M, Tabe T, Nakano K, Fujiwara S, Takao Y, Toda G. Ethanol patch test: a simple method for identifying the effectiveness of cyanamide in alcoholics. Alc Clin Exp Res. 2000 Apr;24(4 Suppl):39S-42S.

with disulfiram (and as with most other drugs too) then provided that Adverse Effects do not intervene, the correct dose is 'enough to cause the desired therapeutic effect'. However, it has not yet been established whether obvious local flushing means that the deterrent effect after a dose of alcohol will be adequate. Some research in this area with disulfiram instead of cyanamide would be welcome and a simple blood test to establish the level of ALDH inhibition might be helpful, although that might not translate directly to the potential severity of the DAR.

Chapter 15. THE ETHICS, PHILOSOPHY AND POLITICS OF DISULFIRAM TREATMENT

For a significant section of the alcoholism treatment community, all pharmacological treatments are inappropriate once any treatment for acute withdrawal symptoms has been completed. In particular, the 12-step movement, which is large and influential in the USA, but smaller and much less influential in Britain, has a long history of opposing medication. A German alcoholism specialist reported that 12-step groups in Germany have a motto that denotes their opposition to all medicines: 'Nichts über die zunge'. It translates as 'nothing over the tongue' and 'nothing' means 'no medication'.[195] This is what makes AA very different from most other self-help groups that exist to give aid and comfort to people suffering from particular conditions. Most self-help groups discuss and disburse information about a range of treatments, trying to protect members from the more obviously useless, harmful or exploitative ones but not usually having Strong Views. They do not, in general, favour one treatment over all evidence-based alternatives, especially for conditions (of which sadly alcoholism is one) in which successful outcomes are by no means certain and relapse or even death cannot always be prevented. AA is more like religions, or organisations that proclaim with unmerited certainty that schizophrenia is caused by vitamin deficiencies and can be cured with mega-vitamin supplements. (If only it

---

[195] Mann K. Personal communication.

were true.) It is also similar to Catholic family-planning agencies which, for doctrinal reasons, will discuss mathematical methods for avoiding unwelcome pregnancy but not mechanical or pharmacological ones.

The founders of AA were much less dogmatic. In 1958, one of them - Bill Wilson - insisted that: "We must also realise that the discoveries of the psychiatrists and the biochemists have vast implications for us alcoholics..... many...patients [have] made good recoveries without AA at all. It should here be noted that some of the recovery methods employed outside AA are quite in contradiction to AA principles and practice. Nevertheless, we of AA ought to applaud the fact that certain of these efforts are meeting with increasing success. ..Therefore, I would like to make a pledge to the whole medical fraternity that AA will always stand ready to cooperate, that AA will never trespass upon medicine, that our members who feel the call will increasingly help in those great enterprises of education, rehabilitation and research which are now going forward with such great promise".[196] That 'increasing success' of the psychiatrists and biochemists has not been very obvious but we can surely commend Bill Wilson's apparent openness to evidence and willingness to cooperate with medicine. This may have been related to the fact that although he managed to abstain from alcohol, he remained addicted to the cigarettes that caused the chronic and eventually fatal obstructive lung disease that made him dependent on both doctors and oxygen, as well as on

---

[196] Lecture to New York Medical Society, 1958. Brown University Digest of Addiction Theory and Application, 13, (5) May 1994, p 12.

barbiturates for sleep. He also used LSD and was said to be a sex addict (and sexual pest) to a degree that embarrassed his colleagues. [197] Wilson's successors were generally antagonistic on both counts.

There is much variation in 12-step groups and some are less dogmatic about disulfiram (and drug treatments in general) than others. I usually encouraged my patients to try AA if they had not already experienced it but when I referred them to the established group based in Westminster Hospital, they reported that if they mentioned that they were taking disulfiram, they were very strongly pressured to stop taking it. In contrast, I once visited a hospital in Ireland where the AA group not only provided its usual group support and 'buddy' system but also ran a rota for supervising disulfiram in patients who were supposed to be taking it. The hospital was situated in a small agricultural town and most of the patients were able either to walk there or to get a lift from someone if they didn't have their own transport. (Some of them drove to the hospital in their tractors.) I thought this was an exemplary arrangement and telephoned AA headquarters in Dublin later to see if they knew of other groups that worked in the same way. There was a rather shocked silence, quickly followed by an assurance that this could not possibly be a proper AA group and that there was certainly nothing like it anywhere else in Ireland. When I returned to London, I visited AA headquarters there to see if

---

[197] Dodes L, Dodes Z. The sober truth. Debunking the bad science behind 12-step programs and the rehab industry. Boston. Beacon. 2015

they would support the setting up of a similar group. They said they would think about it but that was all they ever did.

Not all residential 'rehabs' are run on 12-step lines, though many are. However, it is the almost universal policy of residential clinics or even simple hostels for alcoholics, whatever their philosophy, that if patients drink while they are in residence, they are required to leave. In other words, if they show signs of the problem that was the cause of their admission in the first place, they are denied treatment aimed at modifying that behaviour. This is like telling schizophrenics that if they continue to hallucinate or behave in paranoid ways after admission, they will be discharged. Even outpatient services, or residential establishments with a more tolerant outlook, may not tolerate more than one or two relapses, yet very few of them offer to continue treatment provided the patient will agree to take supervised disulfiram as part of the bargain.

When naltrexone was being studied for its effects in alcoholism, the first attempt to recruit patients through the research institution's 12-step group failed because the group was opposed in principle to medication. A more determined researcher managed to persuade them to give it a try and published the first report. [198] Because naltrexone is moderately effective in reducing drinking but has little effect on abstinence rates, that makes it unattractive to AA groups for whom abstinence is the only acceptable goal. Naltrexone is much more effective in maintaining abstinence when the

---

[198] Kleber H. Personal communication.

drug concerned is an opiate, as discussed later. The increasing evidence that naltrexone depot preparations and implants can have large effects on abstinence rates after opiate withdrawal has made some 12-step clinics and rehabs break with tradition and ideology, but that is a very recent development.

Another group with ambivalent or frankly hostile attitudes are to be found among the numerous non-medical health-professionals working in addiction. The lack of interest in alcoholism displayed by most physicians and psychiatrists for many years allowed the expanding and ambitious professions of clinical psychology, social work and counselling to get a foothold in the specialty. It is understandable that they do not wish to lose it, and that they might see the use of disulfiram and other medications as a threat to their status.

As has been pointed out by authorities such as William Miller [199] and even by AA sympathisers such as Mathew et al, [200] this is particularly true of non-medical professionals working in 12-step establishments, even if they are not 'graduates' of the clinic in question. Mathew et al concede that the emphasis in many clinics in the US and elsewhere on several weeks of profitable inpatient treatment, delivered largely by poorly paid ex-patients trained exclusively in AA ideology, discourages the development of rational, effective, flexible and cost-effective treatment programmes. This may

---

[199] Miller W, Hester R. In-patient alcoholism treatments: who benefits? Am Psychologist 1986;41:794-805.

[200] Mathew RJ, Georgi J, Nagy P. Substance Abuse Treatment: Beyond the Minnesota Model. North Carolina Med J 1994;55:224-6

be one explanation for the surprising results of a survey which revealed that even US addiction physicians prescribed disulfiram or naltrexone for fewer than 15% of their alcoholic patients.[201] Another possible explanation is that in the USA, many addiction physicians are 'recovering addicts' who attribute their recovery to the 12-step philosophy that is still hegemonic in that country. In no other country – at least in our experience - is this kind of physician or this kind of hegemony at all common.

As well as resistance from 12-step clinics originating from both financial and ideological concerns, there are other primarily financial reasons for neglect and under-use. Disulfiram is an old drug, long out of patent protection. It is thus comparatively cheap (particularly in comparison with naltrexone and acamprosate in most countries) and is often marketed by manufacturers of 'generic' drugs who do no advertising and sponsor no research. In contrast to naltrexone and acamprosate, few disulfiram studies in the last forty years have received any funding from disulfiram manufacturers. Given the criticisms that have been levelled at industry-sponsored research, that fact should reinforce the credibility of the overwhelmingly positive outcomes in the studies of supervised disulfiram that have been done. Conversely, the ready availability of pharmaceutical industry funding for naltrexone and acamprosate research means that researchers and departments looking for projects and funding

---

[201] Mark TL, Kranzler HR, Song X, et al. Physicians' opinions about medications to treat alcoholism. Addiction 2003;98:617–26.

are much more likely to study naltrexone or acamprosate than disulfiram. This imbalance should be reversed.

Finally, although psychoanalysis, and its allied cults, is a spent force in many countries, its residual influence – particularly among counsellors - often leads to a search for 'underlying problems', typically 'unconscious', that are alleged to be the cause of the alcoholism and that must be addressed and dealt with if there to be any hope of lasting (or even partial) improvement.

This belief is similar to the dire and unfounded predictions that 'symptom substitution' would inevitably occur if phobias were treated with CBT techniques such as exposure and anxiety management, rather than by the teasing out of Oedipal hangups. It will bear occasional repeating that in practice, many apparently 'underlying' problems are a result rather than a cause of the alcoholism and disappear or improve with amazing rapidity if drinking ceases. As previously noted, any problems that persist despite abstinence can be categorised and dealt with, in whichever way the patient prefers (including Freudian, Jungian, Adlerian and Kleinian ways) much more easily when treatment is not interrupted by frequent relapses. A psychoanalyst would actually be very well placed to supervise disulfiram during all those Monday to Friday 50-minute hours but we find it rather difficult to believe that this has ever happened in the entire hundred-odd-year period since Sigmund Freud stopped regularly and heavily medicating himself with cocaine.[202]

In 2004, an editorial in Addiction conceded that supervised disulfiram is an effective intervention and it was accompanied by several positive commentaries, including one from Fuller,[203] the main author of the largely negative 1986 RCT. Only four years previously, however, Addiction's senior editor, the late Prof Griffith Edwards, had strongly criticised DSF treatment as both unethical and lacking an adequate evidence-base.[204] More recently but before the publication of further substantial meta-analytical evidence for the effectiveness of disulfiram, Zullino et al.[205] and Thorens et al.[206] argued that the use of disulfiram had no theoretical justification. They claimed that its apparent effectiveness in comparative trials against purely psychosocial interventions or against other drugs such as ACP and NTX was an artefact that could be explained without invoking any true pharmacological effects of DSF. Furthermore, they argued

---

[202] Masson J.(Trans.and Ed.).The complete letters of Sigmund Freud to Wilhelm Fliess. Cambridge, MA: Belknap/Harvard. 1985 *passim*.
[203] Fuller R, Gordis E. Does disulfiram have a role in alcoholism treatment today? Addiction 2004;99:21–4.
[204] Edwards G. Alcohol, the ambiguous molecule. London: Penguin. 2000
[205] Zullino D, Wullschleger A, Thorens G, et al. Le disulfirame, un traitement? Soyons logique. Premiere partie: Le disulfirame, peut-il être considéré comme un traitement phamacologique? (Is disulfiram really a treatment? Let's be logical. Can disulfiram be considered a pharmacological treatment. Part 1. Rev Med Suisse 2010:10:565–7.
[206] Thorens G, Manghi R, Khan R, et al. Le disulfirame, un traitement? Soyons logique. Deuxieme partie: Le disulfirame, peut-il être considéré comme un traitement psychologique? (Is disulfiram really a treatment? Let's be logical. Part 2. Can disulfiram be considered a psychological treatment?). Rev Med Suisse 2010;10:584–7.

that because disulfiram treatment involved the threat of an unpleasant experience, it was morally unacceptable and that the use and marketing of disulfiram for alcoholism should end. These criticisms, which were clearly intended to make clinicians feel uncomfortable about using disulfiram, reveal a misunderstanding of the mechanisms by which disulfiram achieves its therapeutic effects. As we have already shown, they are cognitive-behavioural and educational rather than pharmacological or psychopharmacological. We summarise below the principal objections to disulfiram presented by these authors, followed by our responses and comments.

An important but more specific objection held by some disulfiram opponents is that disulfiram treatment involves the threat of 'punishment' and that it is therefore inappropriate for physicians to take part in it. There are a number of possible responses to such objections, including the obvious ones - that treatment is not compulsory and that 'punishment' usually means something unwelcome, unpleasant, and degrading done to a person, usually against their will, by society or individuals. In the case of disulfiram, any unpleasantness is not done by physicians to patients but by patients to themselves and they can easily avoid it. Most disulfiram patients do just that by not drinking, which is after all the usual mutually agreed long-term aim of the treatment. Another response is to regard the use of disulfiram as a matter rather like abortion or contraception, on which good men and women may hold opposing opinions. In such situations, most developed and democratic societies (Eastern as well as Western) allow both patients and doctors to make their own ethical choices and to participate in or refrain from treatment as they think fit.

There are also pharmacological objections. For example, some researchers state: "disulfiram represents a very notable pharmaco-therapeutic anomaly. Normally, we regard a medication as effective if it deploys its pharmacological effect (this being the basis of placebo-controlled trials). However, disulfiram is supposed to be effective when it isn't producing a pharmacological effect."[207] (Our translation.).

While it is true that disulfiram's efficacy is due to a unique mechanism of action, this pharmacological effect has two facets. First, if the mere probability of an unpleasant DAR is a sufficient deterrent, then disulfiram is doing its job. Second, if the patient needs to experience the DAR personally before deterrence reaches adequate levels, then disulfiram is also doing its job. In both cases, the pharmacology of disulfiram is ultimately what causes the deterrent effect.

In our experience and that of other clinicians, it is exceptional for patients to expose themselves repeatedly to a DAR unless an inadequate dose makes the DAR so mild that it has insufficient deterrent effect. If they do test it and experience a sufficiently unpleasant effect, they will only try it once or twice. Rather than expose themselves to it repeatedly, they are more likely to drop out of treatment despite attempts to help them to stay, thereby demonstrating that they are not really willing to accept even a period of

---

[207] Zullino D, et al. *Op. cit.*

abstinence. This avoids much wasted time and effort for both therapist and patient.

It also refutes a common and important misunderstanding about disulfiram - the allegation or implication that it is a variety of 'aversion therapy'. That term has a very specific meaning and involves the repeated pairing of particular stimuli, such as alcohol or certain types of sexual imagery, with an unpleasant response with the aim of establishing a conditioned response that ideally causes a previously desired or habitual behaviour to become a source of disgust or fear.

In contrast, patients treated with disulfiram are not expected to convince themselves that the pleasures they obtained from drinking never existed or that drinking is an intrinsically undesirable or wicked activity. The aim of treatment is not hatred of alcohol but relative indifference to it, so that it no longer occupies a salient place in the patient's thoughts and habits. Just as it is not necessary, in most cases, for drivers to be fined or arrested before their driving behaviour is modified by speed cameras, most patients taking disulfiram do not need to experience the DAR before they modify their drinking behaviour. Being fined, or experiencing a DAR, may reinforce those modifications but they are not essential, whereas in aversion therapy, the repeated experience of an unpleasant response is an essential and defining part of the aversive conditioning process. In disulfiram treatment, the deterrence or prevention of one particular response to alcohol is usually combined with encouragement, training and practice in different and less harmful responses. The fact that some patients successfully treated with disulfiram become controlled drinkers, sometimes with the assistance of intermittent or 'targeted' disulfiram, is further proof that it does not work by producing conditioned aversion.

Opponents also question whether the ritual of taking a tablet is the crucial factor in the decision to drink or abstain, whether or not the tablet contains DSF. That obviously depends on whether the patient is informed as to the composition of the tablet. For example, in an open label study, Chick et al. showed that supervised DSF, even at rather modest doses, is more effective than supervised ascorbic acid, [208] which patients were told might be helpful in some more general and undefined way that did not involve an unpleasant reaction with alcohol.

The final objection of the Geneva group is that the deterrent effect depends on the patient behaving like a rational actor, "able to evaluate the costs and benefits of his choices. But it is precisely the inability to make such evaluations that is the central element in the definition of an addiction". In reality, most addicts have no general "inability" to act rationally. They may react irrationally or inappropriately in relation to alcohol, as spider phobics do to spiders, but the agreed object of treatment, achieved more effectively with disulfiram than without it, is precisely to assist them to act more rationally in alcohol-related situations.

Their ability to act rationally in other situations is not usually in question, otherwise how would a person with a history of

---

[208] Chick J, Gough K, Falkowski W, et al. Disulfiram treatment of alcoholism. Br J Psychiat 1992; 161:84–9.

alcoholism ever gain employment?

The resistance to the deterrence model of treatment may be only one aspect of a more general trend that regards deterrence as inferior to 'positive reinforcement' (i.e. reward) in programmes for changing undesirable behaviour. This position may be politically correct but is not always scientifically correct. According to Shepherd, "Deterrence is an established theme in criminal justice, but its role in prevention of assault has been treated with ambivalence and even hostility in medicine". [209]

Shepherd registered no dissent when it was suggested in published comment that "[Shepherd] seems to be saying that although selective deterrence works rather well, there are influential people in medicine, psychology and criminology who fervently wish that it didn't because its success conflicts with their ideologies". [210]

Discussing the reluctance of educational welfare officers to bring proceedings against truanting children and their families, only three cases having been brought to court in the previous three years, a juvenile court magistrate wrote: "They do not accept that bringing proceedings will be a deterrent to other parents because they do not believe in the principle of deterrence". [211]

---

[209] Shepherd JP. Criminal deterrence as a public health strategy. Lancet 2001; 358:1717–22.
[210] Brewer C. The deterrence issue. Lancet 2002;359:982.
[211] Liversedge M. Beating truancy. Spectator, 15 July1978. 18

Chapter 16. THE IMPLICATIONS OF DISULFIRAM'S EFFECTIVENESS AND MODES OF ACTION FOR THE HYPOTHESIS THAT 'ADDICTION IS A CHRONIC BRAIN DISEASE'

As well as arguments about the place of medication in managing alcoholism, another vigorous current debate revolves around the claim that alcoholism, like other addictions, is a chronic brain disease. This is increasingly the prevailing view among US researchers but it is also quite popular elsewhere. Volkow et al summarise the 'brain disease' model thus. "Although initial experimentation with a drug of abuse is largely a voluntary behavior, continued drug use can eventually impair neuronal circuits in the brain that are involved in free will, turning drug use into an automatic compulsive behavior.... Exposure to the drug, drug cues, or stress results in unrestrained hyperactivation of the motivation/drive circuit that results in the compulsive drug intake that characterizes addiction."[212]

Yet neither the superior effectiveness nor the apparent mode of action of disulfiram appear to involve the action or modification of specific brain reward or craving pathways or their neurophysiological mechanisms. They do not require the postulating of a 'brain disease'. As Gossop has noted, although there is "clear evidence that neuroadaptive changes

---

[212] Volkow, N.D., Wang, G.J., Fowler, J.S., Tomasi, D., Telang, F., and Baler, R. Addiction: decreased reward sensitivity and increased expectation sensitivity conspire to overwhelm the brain's control circuit. Bioessays 32(9):748–755, 2010.

occur in association with addiction [t]hese are not in themselves evidence of 'damage' or of 'disease'. Neuroadaptive changes occur not only after long-term use: they can occur after a single drug exposure and may develop within a few minutes. Neuroscience has revealed the mechanisms of these adaptive changes."[213]

He also points out that habituation, which must be involved in both becoming addicted and ceasing to be so, is "the capacity of a living system to establish a homeostatic equilibrium in response to change produced by external stimuli." It has "been observed in organisms of all evolutionary levels. Furthermore, these changes occur in psychological processes that do not involve drug self-administration, including perception, learning, memory and forgetting (unlearning)."

In other words; "Practically everything in the neurone is somehow involved in addiction, just as it is in other forms of behaviour and adaptation." This may explain how the nervous system works (ie what the 'machinery' is) but "it does not explain how environmental influences affect the operation of this machinery. Nor what directs it to addiction rather than to other behaviours."

Admittedly, Gossop continues, Leshner [214] concedes that

---

[213] Gossop M. Limitations in the clinical use of all this neurobiological knowledge. Invited paper presented at 13th annual meeting International Society of Addiction Medicine. Oslo Sept 2011.
[214] Leshner, A. Addiction is a brain disease, and it matters. Science. 1997 278, 45-7.

addiction is *"not just a brain disease"* while Volkow and Li[215] have stated that the brain disease model should be "combined with new knowledge of how environmental...and developmental factors contribute to addiction". However, "current neurobiological approaches do not explain why (among many epidemiological findings) consumption of alcohol, even by alcoholics, varies with disposable income and ease of availability; why children of alcoholics may become alcoholics (or not) or may become total abstainers; why the prevalence of alcoholism in France fell sharply with changes in public attitudes in the past 20 years; and why the prevalence of heroin and other forms of drug addiction (in Norway, UK, and in almost all countries) is now massively greater than in the relatively recent past: such changes cannot plausibly be attributed to neurobiological factors. The 'brain disease' model also has little to say about such clinical matters as why heroin-addicted US soldiers in Vietnam who became abstinent after treatment in the USA mostly remained abstinent, whereas 'street' addicts who became abstinent during institutional treatment rapidly relapsed on return to former drug-associated environment; or why heroin is largely smoked in the Netherlands but almost exclusively injected in Norway. Furthermore, while synaptic plasticity is one of the important neurochemical foundations of learning and memory, attempts to treat addiction by medications that block activation of the 'reward pathway' have given only modest results."

---

[215] Volkow N., Li T. Drugs and alcohol: treating and preventing abuse, addiction and their medical consequences. Pharmacol Ther. 2005 108,3-17.

We have quoted Gossop so extensively not only because his arguments (first presented at an international conference) are relevant to our hypothesis but also because this major critique of the 'brain disease' model by a very distinguished British addiction researcher has not, at the time of writing, been submitted for publication, though Kalant[216] has made some similar points. Marc Lewis has also strongly criticised the 'brain disease' model of addiction and brings to the debate his own personal experience of heroin addiction.[217] Gossop's comments emphasise especially the failure of the model to explain not only *recovery from addiction*, but the fact that after many years of uninterrupted abuse, recovery can sometimes be instant, lasting and unrelated to treatment.

These points strongly reinforce our conclusion that the mechanism by which disulfiram facilitates the move from alcoholism to lasting abstinence more effectively than other current medications or medication-free programmes, is essentially *educational or psychological* rather than neurobiological or neuropharmacological. Indeed, one of the few studies to examine the contribution of the various components of a comprehensive supervised disulfiram treatment package (albeit for a relatively short period) found that "the contribution of the disulfiram component…was much greater than that of any of the psychotherapeutic components … and that none of the varieties of specific

---

[216] Kalant H. What neurobiology cannot tell us about addiction. Addiction. 2009; 105; 780-9
[217] Lewis M. The biology of desire. Why addiction is not a disease. New York. Public Affairs. 2015, *passim*

psychotherapy was clearly superior to any of the others".[218]

We agree with Gossop, Lewis and several other respected researchers that this neuroplasticity of various brain structures and circuits, which Koob and Volkow[219] appear to regard as neuronal abnormalities underlying the addiction syndrome, can equally be regarded as activities that simply reflect the natural adaptation of the brain to its environment, a process usually called 'learning'. Indeed, all the brain modifications observed in various brain addiction studies might simply reflect the enhancement of synaptic plasticity of NMDA receptors in dopamine neurons in association with drug-associated memories.[220] Repeated exposure to alcohol simply promotes the formation of drug-associated memories. In other words (and to reiterate) it is a learning process and effective treatment involves specific and different learning, re-learning and un-learning processes. Seen in this light, the brain changes observed in developing and recovering from alcoholism are no different in principle from those seen in people who learn a second language [221] (or a musical

---

[218] Carroll KM, Nich C, Ball SA, McCance E. Rounsaville B J. Treatment of cocaine and alcohol dependence with psychotherapy and disulfiram. Addiction 1998;93 (5), 713-728.
[219] Koob GF, Volkow ND. Neurocircuitry of addiction. Neuropsychopharmacol 2010 January; 35(1): 217–238.
[220] Bernier BE, Whitaker LR, Morikawa H. Previous ethanol experience enhances synaptic plasticity of NMDA receptors in the ventral tegmental area. J Neurosci. 2011 April 6; 31(14): 5205–5212.
[221] Mechelli A, Crinion JT, Noppeney U, O'Doherty J, Ashburner J, Frackowiak RS, Price CJ. Neurolinguistics: structural plasticity in the bilingual brain. Nature. 2004 Oct 14;431(7010):757.

instrument [222]) which are changes that are not generally considered as pathological. Comparable changes in relevant cortical areas are seen after purely psychological interventions in a range of psychiatric conditions. [223] The changes that are observed in neuroimaging studies at all stages of alcoholism are largely the results of typical cerebral plasticity associated with a learning process. They are not the result of a brain disease. Truly neuropathological changes may result from the toxic effects of drugs (most notably alcohol) but they are usually transient and, unless severe, not clearly related to long-term outcome.

Even if some brain changes or abnormalities predate alcohol abuse and reflect genetic differences that may make some individuals more vulnerable to various addictions, genes are not destiny. There appear to be genuine genetic factors affecting the risk of alcoholism, at least in men, but I have taken histories from many non-alcoholic patients with a strong family history of alcoholism. They often say: 'I saw what alcohol did to my father and I swore never to touch it'. In any case, disulfiram seems to have the same deterrent effects in patients with and without a family history.

Recovery from alcoholism, however it is defined, involves learning new patterns of behaviour and cognition that not only become progressively easier to practise with time but also increasingly automatic. Relapse in alcoholism means,

---

[222] Lappe C, Herholz SC, Trainor LJ, Pantev C. Cortical plasticity induced by short-term unimodal and multimodal musical training. J Neurosci. 2008 Sep 24;28(39):9632-9.
[223] Linden DE. How psychotherapy changes the brain--the contribution of functional neuroimaging. Mol Psychiatry. 2006 Jun;11(6):528-38.

among other things, the interruption of that process. However, what distinguishes relapse in the treatment of alcoholism (and indeed all types of substance abuse) from other interruptions in a learning process is that by definition, it involves not simply a reversion to behaviours mutually agreed by the therapist/teacher and the patient/pupil to be counter-productive and undesirable. It also typically involves intoxication for a period of hours, days or weeks, during which the patient's ability to respond to rational argument, to regain control, or even to discuss the situation, is severely impaired or absent. This impairment may be aggravated by the 'abstinence violation effect'.[224]

Comparison with other learning processes also helps us to understand why disulfiram is so much more efficient than pharmacotherapies that target specific brain systems. Students can learn a second language from a book without help, just as patients may improve without treatment. However, a teacher can help students to be more regular and efficient in their learning techniques. The similarity with psychotherapies is obvious, though in both settings, large and positive non-specific and placebo effects may contribute to a good outcome. In programmes that include disulfiram, the combination of an effective relapse-preventing medication with the need for regular – if usually brief - contact with the therapeutic team provides in-built opportunities for advice about the psycho-social components of treatment. For

---

[224]Walton MA, Castro FG, Barrington EH. The role of attributions in abstinence, lapse, and relapse following substance abuse treatment. Addict Behav. 1994 May-Jun;19(3):319-31.

example, Garland et al.[225] showed that abstinent alcohol dependent patients commonly use the possibly counterproductive technique of thought-suppression to cope with intrusive cognitions about alcohol, thus inadvertently biasing attention towards alcohol-related stimuli. Like a good French teacher, simple monitoring and advice could assist them to avoid unhelpful learning techniques of this kind.

---

[225] Garland EL, Franken IH, Sheetz JJ, Howard MO. Alcohol attentional bias is associated with autonomic indices of stress-primed alcohol cue-reactivity in alcohol-dependent patients. Exp Clin Psychopharmacol. 2012 Jun;20(3):225-35.

Chapter 17. DISULFIRAM vs OTHER MEDICATIONS FOR ALCOHOLISM

Several post-2000 meta-analyses have concluded that supervised disulfiram is more effective than acamprosate or naltrexone and none has found it less effective. Some of these conclusions are based on comparative trials while others are based on treatment effect sizes. Although the superiority of disulfiram is important when considering the choice of treatment, both the meta-analyses and the effect size studies probably underestimate the degree of superiority. The reason is that in most studies of disulfiram, the prescribed doses would have been inadequate for a significant proportion of patients who risked drinking, as some always do. Since these patients thereby qualify for a 'difficult' label, outcomes would probably have been even better if their doses had been increased, as happened in several studies and case-histories.[226,227,228] when the DAR was initially absent or inadequate. While some patients might drop out of treatment at higher doses because of extreme ambivalence about becoming abstinent even for a while, it seems very likely, as we have argued previously, that a useful

---

[226] Bickel WK, Rizzuto P, Zielony RD, Klobas J, Pangiosonlis P, Mernit R, Knight WF. Combined Behavioral and Pharmacological Treatment of Alcoholic Methadone Patients. J Subst Abuse. 1988-1989;1(2):161-71.

[227] Brewer C. Long-term, high-dose disulfiram in the treatment of alcohol abuse. Brit J Psychiat 1993;163:687-9

[228] Newton-Howes G, Levack WM, McBride S, Gilmor M, Tester R. Non-physiological mechanisms influencing disulfiram treatment of alcohol use disorder: A grounded theory study. Drug Alc Depend 2016;165:126-31.

proportion would have persevered and thus resumed abstinence.

In contrast there is no clinical evidence that increasing the dose of either naltrexone or acamprosate beyond the standard recommended levels (other than in very obese patients) would improve outcomes in patients who had continued to drink heavily despite taking those medications. In a few cases, it is possible that the symbolism of an increased dose might improve the placebo effect of medication but it would not improve the pharmacological effect, which is very modest and not always visible. Mann et al, noting that: "The results of placebo-controlled trials (RCTs) with acamprosate or naltrexone vary substantially" did a well-controlled comparison of those two drugs with placebo and added "biweekly manualised 'medical management' to enhance compliance" so as to compare their results with those of the similar but much larger COMBINE study in the US. They found that for the main outcome measure - time until the first occurrence of heavy drinking - "neither acamprosate nor naltrexone [supplied] any additional benefit compared with placebo".[229] COMBINE itself had not provided much excuse for therapeutic rejoicing. "Acamprosate showed no significant effect on drinking vs placebo" while "patients receiving naltrexone plus medical management, Combined

---

[229] Mann K, Lemenager T, Hoffmann S, Reinhard I, Hermann D, Batra A, Berner M, Wodarz N, Heinz A, Smolka MN, Zimmermann US, Wellek S, Kiefer F, Anton RF. Results of a double-blind, placebo-controlled pharmacotherapy trial in alcoholism conducted in Germany and comparison with the US COMBINE study. Addict Biol. 2013 Nov;18(6):937-46.

Behavioral Intervention (CBI) plus Medical Management and placebos, or both naltrexone and CBI plus medical management, had higher percent days abstinent (80.6, 79.2, and 77.1, respectively)" compared with other combinations of management and active or placebo medication.[230] These clinically insignificant differences between naltrexone and placebo occurred despite patients receiving 100mg/day of naltrexone, instead of the usual 50mg.

Perhaps because these small differences between naltrexone and placebo were so disappointing, Oslin et al[231] explored the potentially exculpatory suggestion that "functional polymorphism (rs1799971, Asn40Asp) of the µ-opioid receptor gene (OPRM1) is associated with the risk of relapse to heavy drinking following treatment with the opioid antagonist naltrexone". Sadly, they found that in a placebo-controlled trial of naltrexone 50mg/day, "A significant reduction in heavy drinking occurred across all groups (P = .001). Other drinking outcomes, and all secondary outcomes, demonstrated similar time effects, with no genotype × treatment interaction." Again, the difference between active and placebo groups was modest.

---

[230] Anton RF, O'Malley SS, Ciraulo DA, Cisler RA, Couper D, Donovan DM, Gastfriend DR, Hosking JD, Johnson BA, LoCastro JS, Longabaugh R, Mason BJ, Mattson ME, Miller WR, Pettinati HM, Randall CL, Swift R, Weiss RD, Williams LD, Zweben A; COMBINE Study Research Group. Combined pharmacotherapies and behavioral interventions for alcohol dependence: the COMBINE study: a randomized controlled trial. JAMA. 2006 May 3;295(17):2003-17.
[231] Oslin DW, Leong SH, Lynch KG, Berrettini W, O'Brien CP, Gordon AJ, Rukstalis M. Naltrexone vs Placebo for the Treatment of Alcohol Dependence: A Randomized Clinical Trial. JAMA Psychiatry. 2015 May;72(5):430-7

Even 100% compliance with a relatively ineffective medication will not greatly improve the outcome in placebo comparisons. Since injections have more powerful placebo effects than tablets, we would expect better results than with oral medication but treatment outcomes in alcoholism with depot naltrexone are not very much better than outcomes with placebo injections. In one of the placebo-controlled trials of depot naltrexone[232] that preceded the granting of a product licence in the USA, the placebo injection was only 25% less effective than the active injection by one measure. Several patients continued to drink heavily despite being on a full dose of active medication – something that almost never happens with disulfiram. Unsurprisingly, patients who had managed to become abstinent before starting medication had better outcomes than those who did not, in both active and placebo groups. That rather suggests that patients with milder forms of alcohol dependence were more likely to be helped than those with severe alcoholism.

Most patients in this trial of injectable naltrexone were not daily heavy drinkers. The average monthly number of heavy drinking days, defined as more than four US standard drinks daily, was 14 to 15. Few patients seem to have been consuming more than the equivalent of a bottle of wine on

---

[232] Garbutt JC, Kranzler HR, O'Malley SS, Gastfriend DR, Pettinati HM, Silverman BL, Loewy JW, Ehrich EW. Efficacy and tolerability of long-acting injectable naltrexone for alcohol dependence: a randomized controlled trial. JAMA. 2005 Apr 6;293(13):1617-25.

their drinking days. In another study[233] using a slightly lower dose of depot naltrexone, around 80% of the patients had either not had any previous treatment for alcoholism or had only one previous treatment. Only 5% in the naltrexone group needed any kind of detoxification from alcohol before starting treatment, again suggesting relatively moderate drink problems. The patients in this study sound very different from alcoholics who drink the equivalent of a bottle of spirits or more every day, have badly damaged their physical health as well as their social and family relationships, and need in-patient treatment for withdrawal (like many of the OLITA patients) yet these more challenging patients are common in alcoholism services. It remains to be demonstrated whether such preparations will be as effective as supervised disulfiram in recurrent alcohol-related offenders. We strongly suspect that they will not.

When treatment effect sizes are examined, the advantage of depot naltrexone over a placebo injection also appears marginal. In a trial where analysis by treatment group "showed no significant effect", NTX subjects reported a mean of 22.4 days of heavy drinking during the study period, compared with 25.3 days for placebo group. The effect size for this difference was 0.12, which - as the authors of the trial admitted - is "in the small range of effect sizes." A Swedish meta-analysis was slightly more generous to both naltrexone and acamprosate, awarding them average treatment effect

---

[233] Kranzler H, Wesson D, Billot L. Naltrexone depot for treatment of alcohol dependence: a multicenter, randomized, placebo-controlled clinical trial. Alc Clin Exp Res. 2004 Jul;28(7):1051-9.

sizes of 0.28 and 0.26 respectively. The figure for supervised disulfiram was 0.53.[234] Even imperfect compliance with a highly effective medication may produce good results and improving that level of compliance will produce even better ones.

As Skinner et al's 2014 meta-analysis noted, fair direct comparisons of disulfiram with other drugs can only be done in open controlled trials. The first published randomised controlled study comparing supervised naltrexone and supervised disulfiram in pure alcoholism showed that disulfiram was significantly more effective, even though – intriguingly – the naltrexone patients reported somewhat lower craving levels.[235] The differences were not just statistically significant; they were really striking and clinically important. After 12 months, nearly twice as many patients were relapse-free on disulfiram - 86% - as on NTX - 44% - (a very impressive[236] p=0.0009). Survival time until the first relapse to heavy drinking was longer with disulfiram (119 vs 63 days p=0.020); and gamma-glutamate

---

[234] Berglund M, Thelander S, Salaspuro M, Franck J, Andréasson S, Öjehagen A. Treatment of Alcohol Abuse: An Evidence-Based Review. Alc Clin Exp Res. 27:1645-1656, 2003)

[235] De Sousa A & de Sousa A. Naltrexone vs disulfiram A one year follow up of alcohol dependence treatment. Alcohol Alcohol. 2004 Nov-Dec;39(6):528-31

[236] *p* (for *probability*) is a standard index of statistical significance. A *p* of <0.05 means a >95% probability that the result was not due to chance. This is the standard *minimal* level of significance but statistical significance does not necessarily translate into clinical significance. Compared with a *p* of just under 0.05 (e.g. 0.049) a *p* of 0.0001 is *490 times* more significant and thus *490 times* less likely to be a chance finding.

transpeptidase (GGT) [237] fell significantly (p=0.038) more than in the NTX group.

The same authors carried out a similar study comparing disulfiram and acamprosate, except that it lasted eight months instead of twelve.[238] It produced very similar results. At the end of the trial, 93 of 100 patients were still in contact. If it happened, relapse (the consumption of >5 drinks/40g of alcohol in one day) occurred at a mean of 123 days with disulfiram compared to 71 days with acamprosate (p = 0.0001). Perhaps more important for patients with serious alcoholism, 88% of patients on disulfiram remained abstinent compared to 46% with acamprosate (p=0.0002). However, as with the naltrexone study, patients allocated to acamprosate had lower craving than those on disulfiram (p=0.002). These anti-craving effects are of both theoretical and practical, therapeutic interest. Theoretical, because understanding – and possibly modifying - the neurophysiology and psychology of craving is an obvious focus of addiction research; practical-therapeutic because in the case of naltrexone, its supposedly general anti-craving effect does not, by itself, seem to translate into more than very modest improvement in outcomes, if that. The failure to find any specific effect of depot-naltrexone on methamphetamine abuse[239] is only the

---

[237] Note for the unmedical. GGT is the standard, basic LFT marker of excessive drinking.

[238] De Sousa A & de Sousa A. An open randomized study comparing disulfiram and acamprosate in the treatment of alcohol dependence. Alcohol Alcohol. 2005 Nov-Dec;40(6):545-8.

[239] Coffin PO, Santos GM, Hern J, Vittinghoff E, Santos D, Matheson T, Colfax G, Batki SL. Extended-Release Naltrexone for Methamphetamine Dependence among Men Who Have Sex with Men: A Randomized

most recent of several negative findings for drugs other than alcohol. These modest or undetectable impacts of naltrexone in the real world of addiction treatment reinforce the doubts that we and others have expressed about the practical value of the 'addiction-as-brain-disease' paradigm – so far, at least.

A similar randomised study comparing disulfiram with both naltrexone and acamprosate was done in Helsinki. Finland is the home of the so-called Sinclair Method of alcoholism treatment with intermittent or 'targeted' naltrexone, in which NTX is not taken daily but only before situations where personal experience suggests a high-risk of drinking too much. As described in the chapter on controlled drinking, disulfiram can be used in a very similar way.

Unsurprisingly, "all three study groups showed marked reduction in drinking, from baseline to the end of the study. During the continuous [partially supervised] medication phase, treatment with disulfiram was more effective in reducing Heavy Drinking Days (HDD) and average weekly alcohol consumption, and increasing time to the first drink, as well as the number of abstinent days. During the TM [unsupervised, Targeted Medication] period, there were no significant differences between the groups in time to first HDD and days to first drinking, but the abstinence days were significantly more frequent in the disulfiram group than acamprosate and naltrexone". [240] This superiority of

---

Placebo-Controlled Trial. Addiction. 22 July 2017 DOI: 10.1111/add.13950
[240] Laaksonen E, Koski-Jännes A, Salaspuro M, Ahtinen H, Alho H. A randomized, multicentre, open-label, comparative trial of disulfiram,

disulfiram occurred even though the 200mg/day dose was not increased if patients continued drinking. The title of a large German study – 'Why is disulfiram superior to acamprosate in the routine clinical setting?' - hardly needs any further comment.[241]

Earlier, a small study had shown that naltrexone had no useful effect in patients who abused both alcohol and cocaine but disulfiram considerably reduced the consumption of both drugs.[242] That was confirmed in a larger study[243] that unexpectedly found disulfiram to be useful for cocaine problems even when alcohol abuse was not an issue. Yet arguably the most striking finding of the study came from its comparison, with and without supervised disulfiram, of two common psychotherapeutic interventions (Cognitive-Behavioural Therapy and Twelve-Step Facilitation) with ordinary clinical management, which acted as a 'minimal psychotherapy' control. Subjects assigned to disulfiram were retained in treatment significantly longer than those assigned to no medication (average 8.4 versus 5.8 weeks, p<0.05). The psychotherapy components actually had little effect on

---

naltrexone and acamprosate in the treatment of alcohol dependence. Alcohol Alcohol. 2008 Jan-Feb;43(1):53-61.
[241] Diehl A, Ulmer L, Mutschler J, Herre H, Krumm B, Croissant B, Mann K, Kiefer F. Why is disulfiram superior to acamprosate in the routine clinical setting? A retrospective long-term study in 353 alcohol-dependent patients. Alcohol Alcohol. 2010 May-Jun;45(3):271-7.
[242] Carroll KM, Ziedonis D, O'Malley S et al. Pharmacologic interventions for abusers of alcohol and cocaine: a pilot study of disulfiram versus naltrexone. Amer J Addict 1993;2:77-79.
[243] Carroll KM, Nich C, Ball SA, McCance E. & Rounsaville B J. Treatment of cocaine and alcohol dependence with psychotherapy and disulfiram. Addiction 1998;93 (5), 713-728.

treatment retention and no significant differences between the two types of psychotherapy were found. "Effect sizes for disulfiram compared with no medication on duration of abstinence from cocaine, alcohol and both were, respectively, 0.42, 0.68 and 0.46." A treatment effect size of 0.68 has a significant clinical impact and is far from marginal. In contrast, "Effect sizes for the active psychotherapies compared with minimal (or placebo) psychotherapy on the duration of abstinence were 0.16 for cocaine, 0.11 for alcohol and 0.18 for both cocaine and alcohol".[244] A treatment effect size of 0.11 is barely visible.

I end this chapter with a comment from a patient who was being visited in his hospital room in the early 1990s. He had previously abstained from heroin for several months with a series of naltrexone implants but he had a short relapse when he discontinued them and had been readmitted for further detoxification and implantation. During the visit, I took a telephone call from a national British newspaper. The use of naltrexone in alcoholism had just made headlines and the newspaper wanted to know more. The patient listened attentively to the conversation. 'Tell them', he said, 'that I drank like a fish when I was on naltrexone'. That may have been an exaggeration because he had never turned up to an appointment drunk and he was a well-mannered and sociable young man who sensibly sought treatment for his heroin abuse before he was due to inherit a large sum of money on his 25th birthday. He had many friends and his drinking was

---

[244] Brewer C. Supervised disulfiram is more effective in alcoholism than naltrexone or acamprosate - or even psychotherapy: How it works and why it matters. Adicciones. 2005. 17(4); 285-96

probably more social than pathological but it was clearly heavy at times and even a naltrexone implant did not impede it.

Chapter 18. WHY CAN'T WE HAVE A DISULFIRAM IMPLANT?

As two of disulfiram's leading pharmacological researchers noted: "For any drug which has to be taken daily on a chronic basis and for which compliance is a problem, administration in depot form as an implant is an obvious solution."[245] We have briefly referred in several previous chapters to the use of implants containing disulfiram that have no enzyme inhibiting effect but which have powerful placebo effects that assist some patients to remain abstinent for lengthy periods. Just as injected placebos have more powerful effects than placebo tablets, so implants or depot injections may have even stronger placebo effects than ordinary injections. However, an implant or depot injection of disulfiram or of a drug with similar ALDH-inhibiting properties would improve outcomes in alcoholism treatment in exactly the same way that implants and depot injections of naltrexone have improved outcomes in the treatment of opiate abuse.

Long-acting preparations of naltrexone are particularly useful for helping recently detoxified opiate abusers through the difficult transition from the psychological and pharmacological comforts of regular use, the loss of those comforts and their replacement by physical and psychological withdrawal symptoms, through to the acceptance and normalization of a new set of cognitive attitudes and behavioural responses to opiates. In all long-term follow-up studies of alcoholism, the length of previous

---

[245] Gessner P, Gessner N. Disulfiram and its metabolites. Buffalo, 1992.

abstinence is one of the best predictors of the length (and likelihood) of future abstinence. This is in line with our suggested analogy between the most effective and efficient ways of learning a new language, which involve consistent and uninterrupted practice for a sufficient period, and of learning and perfecting new and non-drinking responses to alcohol.

For many years, a French (or possibly Swiss) company produced an implantable version of disulfiram called 'Esperal'. More recently, disulfiram implants were produced by a Polish company, Polpharm, but they could not give me any information about blood levels or measures of ALDH inhibition. We do not know who manufactured the implants studied by Johnsen and Mørland in the early 1990s, mentioned earlier, but they were presumably similar to other commercial (if unlicensed) preparations and we do know that they had no pharmacological effects on alcohol metabolism. Implanted patients presumably believed that they would get a DAR if they consumed alcohol and most were deterred by that belief but the researchers showed that the implants did not inhibit ALDH. Indeed, they could not detect disulfiram or its metabolites in blood and when implanted patients were given alcohol slowly and intravenously without their realizing it, no DAR occurred.

Though the negligible amounts of disulfiram released by implants are far too small to produce measurable ALDH inhibition, let alone a significant DAR, they can be large enough to cause fulminant hepatitis in patients predisposed by nickel sensitivity or other factors. A case report from

Hanover[246] described a 35-year old man with a history of alcoholism who had been admitted with jaundice and "a massive increase in aspartate aminotransferase (60,620 Units/l) [normal 10-40], alanine aminotransferase (16,726 Units/l) [normal 7-56], lactate dehydrogenase (38,180 U/l) [normal c.100-300], [gamma]glutamate dehydrogenase (12,211 U/l) [normal 11-50] total bilirubin (179 mmol/l) [normal 3-25]"[247] three days after the end of his latest alcohol binge. Not surprisingly, the liver problems were initially attributed to alcohol but although his liver was enlarged, there was no evidence of cirrhosis or the typical fatty infiltration of alcoholic liver disease and abnormal LFTs in alcoholism usually produce three-figure elevations rather than four- or five-figure ones as in this case. Transferred to intensive care in early hepatic coma, liver transplantation was being considered when further questioning about a small scar on his buttock revealed that he had had a disulfiram implant inserted in Poland two months previously. It had clearly had no effect on his drinking but was almost certainly the cause of the hepatic failure. It was removed and he left intensive care six days later with his liver functions rapidly returning to normal and no lasting damage.

The main reason that DSF implants have no pharmacological effect is that in order to be pharmacologically effective, they would have to be very large. Most people need daily doses of at least 200mg to get a DAR. At that dose, an implant would

---

[246] Meier M, Woywodt A, Hoeper M. Acute liver failure: a message found under the skin Postgrad Med J 2005;81:269–270.
[247] Note for the unmedical: in addition to GGT, these are markers of general, rather than specifically alcoholic, liver dysfunction.

need to contain 6g – 6000mg – of disulfiram to last even a month. In the 1980s and early 1990s, Michael Phillips, a physician with a wide range of research interests, experimented with various subcutaneous suspensions of disulfiram[248] and measured both CS_2 in breath and the effects of test doses of alcohol.[249] There was modest subjective and objective evidence of a DAR for 2-4 weeks but the results were of theoretical rather than practical interest. A few years ago at an international conference, I encountered a physician from Russia who tried to interest me in a 'long acting injection' of disulfiram and produced a pre-loaded 5ml syringe containing an intriguing pink liquid. It contained, he said 250mg of disulfiram. Asked about disulfiram blood levels, he replied: "We cannot detect it but we know it is there"!

If, instead of disulfiram, drug manufacturers would take an interest in its much more potent active metabolite S-methyl N,N-diethylthiolcarbamate sulfoxide, they would find it relatively simple to produce a pharmacologically effective implant. Furthermore, the release characteristics could be tailored so that progressive dose increases could be achieved if the standard dose failed to produce a DAR. Prof Morris Faiman of Kansas University has shown that such an implant can be made. It is formed of biodegradable plastic

---

[248] Phillips M. Persistent sensitivity to ethanol following a single dose of parenteral sustained-release disulfiram. Adv Alcohol Subst Abuse. 1987;7(1):51-61.

[249] Phillips M, Greenberg J. Dose-ranging study of depot disulfiram in alcohol abusers. Alc Clin Exp Res. 1992 Oct;16(5):964-7.

impregnated with the active metabolite[250] and is similar in appearance, size and mode of insertion to long-acting contraceptive implants. Unlike naltrexone, a depot injection of disulfiram would not be acceptable because as the case history above shows, its very rare and idiosyncratic but very serious liver toxicity requires a formulation that would allow it to be quickly, totally and easily removed if necessary. The active metabolite cannot be presumed to be safer than the parent drug in this respect. Unfortunately, the cost of bringing new drugs – or even new formulations of old drugs – to the market is now so high as to discourage products that do not promise large and rapid returns on investment.

The same therapeutic strategies underlying disulfiram and naltrexone implants will be relevant when vaccines or monoclonal antibodies against specific drugs of abuse become available. They will deter use of the drug in question by making it pointless so that eventually, not using may become the automatic default position. 'Alcohol is the main exception to the vaccine approach because it is by far the least potent of all drugs of abuse, for most of which individual doses are measured in milligrammes or even microgrammes. Even cocaine is only consumed in quantities of one or two grammes at a time. This means that the antibodies to these drugs can also be effective at similar dose levels. In contrast, most drinkers need to consume at least

---

[250] Ningaraj NS, Schloss JV, Williams TD, Faiman MD. Glutathione carbamoylation with S-methyl N,N-diethylthiolcarbamate sulfoxide and sulfone. Mitochondrial low Km aldehyde dehydrogenase inhibition and implications for its alcohol-deterrent action. Biochem Pharmacol. 1998;55(6):749-56.

20g of alcohol before they experience significant effects and most alcoholics need two or three times that amount. Even if an antibody to alcohol could be created, the doses required to neutralise it would be prohibitively large

HISTORICAL FOOTNOTE.

The alcoholic former footballer George Best was under the care of a leading London liver specialist in the early 2000s and it was reported in the press that he had received an Antabuse implant. This worried me because over the years, a few patients made their way to my clinic begging me to put in an implant, either because they had had one before (usually in South Africa) and stayed dry, or they had read about them and thought it would solve their problem. Knowing that the implants had a powerful placebo effect and not wanting to disappoint the patients, or to see them end up in the hands of less scrupulous practitioners, I worked out what I think was an acceptable solution to the ethical dilemma. It involved referring them to a cosmetic surgeon who agreed to implant subcutaneously a suitably shaped piece of silicone while repeating the word 'Antabuse' at frequent intervals and assuring the patient that its effects would last for six months, which was what most of them seemed to believe.

This relieved me of ethical anxiety about charging patients for a placebo procedure, though admittedly it simply passed the ethical problem down the road. The number of patients involved was small – fewer than a dozen - but their outcome was rather good. It is a pity that, for obvious reasons, the surgeon and I were not able to write up these results and even if we had tried, I doubt whether any respectable journal would have accepted the paper.

Chapter 19. DISULFIRAM, THE JAPANESE (AGAIN) AND THE POTENTIAL OF GENE THERAPY

Since disulfiram works by reversibly turning alcoholic patients into the equivalent of Japanese ALDH2*2 homozygotes, it has occurred to some researchers that similar results might be obtained more reliably and without the need for regular supervised medication by changing their ALDH genotype into the 'inefficient' variety. Gene therapy is now an established technique for some rare and otherwise untreatable conditions and the basic idea is not very complicated. You find a harmless virus, insert the new, desirable gene into it and inject the modified virus into the patient. If the transfer is successful, the new gene then replaces the old and depending on the technique used, the replacement can be either temporary or permanent.

Gene therapy for alcoholism has not yet been tried on humans[251] but it works quite well for rats. Using specially bred alcohol-preferring rodents known collectively (and delightfully) as 'University of Chile bibulous rats', a group in Santiago have been transferring "therapeutic genes that can modify the expression of disease predisposing genes, an effect that can last from months to years. In line with the above, we have tested if inhibiting the expression of the aldehyde dehydrogenase gene (ALDH2) by an anti-ALDH2 antisense gene can curtail the drive of alcohol-dependent

---

[251] Israel Y. Personal communication

animals to consume alcohol."[252] The bibulous rats were fond enough of alcohol even in their normal state. When allowed to become physically dependent and then deprived of alcohol for three days, so that they suffered the rodent equivalent of the shakes, they were then re-exposed to alcohol. There is evidently also a rat equivalent of the 'hair of the dog' and the now tremulous as well as bibulous creatures drank even more – "ten times higher than…naïve rats". The single injection "reduced liver ALDH2 activity by 85% ($p < 0.002$) and inhibited voluntary ethanol intake by 50% (ANOVA $p < 0.005$) for 34 days".

In the chapter on the Japanese factor, we mentioned that a very small number of ALDH2*2 homozygotes did not have total protection against alcoholism and we discussed the possibility that lower acetaldehyde production because of inefficient *alcohol* dehydrogenase (ADH) might explain it. In a second study, the same group therefore transferred both a *more efficient* version of ADH, to increase acetaldehyde production and a *less efficient* version of ALDH, to increase acetaldehyde levels by reducing its further metabolism.[253] "Animals administered AdV-ADH/asALDH2 showed a 176% increase in liver ADH activity, whereas liver ALDH2 activity was reduced by 24%, and upon the administration of a dose of ethanol (1 g/kg, i.p.), these showed arterial

---

[252] Ocaranza P, Quintanilla ME, Tampier L, Karahanian E, Sapag A, Israel Y. Gene therapy reduces ethanol intake in an animal model of alcohol dependence. Alc Clin Exp Res. 2008 Jan;32(1):52-7.

[253] Rivera-Meza M, Quintanilla ME, Tampier L. Reduction of ethanol consumption in alcohol-preferring rats by dual expression gene transfer. Alcohol Alcohol. 2012 Mar-Apr;47(2):102-8

acetaldehyde levels that were 400% higher than those of animals administered AdV-C. Rats that received the AdV-ADH/asALDH2 vector *reduced by 60% their voluntary ethanol intake versus controls*." (my italics) In other words, even though ALDH activity was reduced less in the second study than in the first, this dual tinkering with alcohol-metabolising genes and enzymes still reduced alcohol consumption considerably. There is, incidentally, no evidence that Japan's atypical gene distribution makes alcoholic liver disease commoner in Japan than elsewhere.[254]

Gene therapy for alcoholism is presumably many years away but it is interesting (and significant) that its most promising manifestation relies on the same principles as disulfiram treatment. Not surprisingly, the Chilean research has caught the attention of the occasional industrious journalist. One account gives a reasonably low-key and factual summary but notes the similarity with disulfiram and makes the usual alarmist mistake of claiming that "The trace of alcohol in mouthwash is enough to trigger a reaction".[255]

---

[254] Lonardo A, Ballestri S, Romagnoli D, Nascimbeni F. Alcohol and Steatosis: The Japanese Paradox. EBioMedicine. 2016;8:23-24
[255] Davison A. Gene Therapy for Alcoholics. An interesting approach to curbing alcoholism is tested on rats. MIT Review. 2008, January 9th

Although Listerine apparently contains about as much alcohol as sherry, it is probably denatured, industrial alcohol – the same as in methylated spirits – and is apparently favoured as a beverage only by the desperate. Most mouthwashes contain less alcohol or none and even with Listerine, merely rinsing the mouth for a few seconds would hardly register. However, researchers in Florida went to the trouble of measuring alcohol and its metabolites in urine and hair in a group of volunteers who gargled with Listerine "four times daily for 3¼ days". In all cases, urine alcohol was at negligible levels but no doubt Listerine aficionados taking disulfiram would be well advised to spit rather than swallow the stuff.[256]

---

[256] Reisfield GM, Goldberger BA, Pesce AJ, Crews BO, Wilson GR, Teitelbaum SA, Bertholf RL. Ethyl glucuronide, ethyl sulfate, and ethanol in urine after intensive exposure to high ethanol content mouthwash. J Anal Toxicol. 2011 Jun;35(5):264-8.

Chapter 20. CONCLUSION

As well as the consistently positive evidence from meta-analyses since 2000, some of the best arguments for using disulfiram come from patients themselves. Disulfiram protects them not only against relapse but also against the endless internal arguments about drinking or not drinking that are one of the daily burdens of alcoholics, especially early in treatment. Remember the patients who described those burdens as a sort of "incessant internal homunculus that demanded alcohol"? Disulfiram replaced the endless ruminations and temptations with a mind-set where "alcohol is simply no longer an option". Remember the patient who described how, when he wasn't taking disulfiram, he was always trying not to drink "but at the end of it, I just go 'fuck it, fuck it'... When I'm on Antabuse, it's just like. Well, I can't". And that "Somewhat counter-intuitively, rather than restricting decision-making autonomy, *choosing to take disulfiram was described by many participants as empowering or even liberating. Disulfiram gave back control over life events by removing the weight of continued rumination on drinking and drinking decisions"*. (our italics) Another patient stated: "I didn't realise what a positive step it was to empower me, to give me some strength back... something to build on. ...Rather than abstinence being a half-hearted commitment – a decision with shifting boundaries – disulfiram made the decision not to drink absolute....". If patients are not spending half their time or more thinking about whether or not to have a drink, it means they have more time to think about the more helpful and constructive things that are crucial for recovery.

No reader who has got this far should think we are suggesting that adding disulfiram to a treatment programme makes treating alcoholism a simple matter with guaranteed high success rates. Only the more shameless 'celebrity rehabs' make suggestions like that. However, the evidence shows clearly and unequivocally that when properly, consistently and rationally used and when integrated with appropriate psycho-social interventions where necessary, disulfiram can greatly improve short-term, medium-term and long-term outcomes. It also shows that disulfiram can make it much easier to manage patients who would be regarded even by experienced clinicians as challenging or 'difficult'; and that it is considerably more effective than the main alternative drugs. Many patients with relatively mild alcoholism and little or no previous treatment do not need medication but when the problem is more serious, or when previous treatment has not been very helpful, then disulfiram is more likely to be helpful than other drugs and should certainly be considered if those drugs are not working.

The common tendency to regard disulfiram as a dangerous drug is alarmist even as a generalization; doubly so when disulfiram's really rather average level of adverse effects is compared with the real, common and lethal dangers of unchecked alcohol abuse. At a conservative estimate, in England alone alcoholism is an important factor in half a million hospital admissions and kills around 15,000 people every year.[257] That is about three times the number of people

---

[257] http://www.lape.org.uk/downloads/AlcoholAttributableFractions.pdf

who commit suicide (quite a few of whom are also alcohol abusers) but the effectiveness of properly supervised disulfiram in alcoholism is much greater than that of pharmacological treatment for depression. As we have discussed, while the evidence-base for disulfiram is strengthening, that for antidepressants is weakening and increasingly questioned. Yet as Suh et al note: "…disulfiram is currently being underused or used in short durations in the United States, given the prevalence of alcoholism. In 1999, there were only 246,000 disulfiram prescriptions written for the treatment of alcoholism in the United States. This rate of prescribing disulfiram for treating alcoholism, which is a disorder that is far more prevalent than depression and schizophrenia, is relatively low and illustrates how disulfiram is proportionally underused when compared with the use of antidepressants and antipsychotics, at 23,138,000 and 6,662,000 prescriptions per year, respectively".[258] In 2012, only 5.1% of nearly 300,000 alcohol-abusing patients seen in the US Veterans Administration health service received any of the medications licensed for alcoholism.[259]

It is not just the effectiveness but also the *cost-effectiveness* of alcoholism treatments which include disulfiram that needs emphasising. Many patients don't require admission and can

---

[258] Suh JJ, Helen M. Pettinati HM, Kampman K, and Charles P. O'Brien CP. The status of disulfiram a half of a century later. J Clin Psychopharmacol 2006:26;3, 290-302

[259] Williams E, Gupta S, Rubinsky A, Glass J, Jones-Webb R, Bensley K, Harris A. Variation in receipt of pharmacotherapy for alcohol use disorders across racial/ethnic groups: A national study in the U.S. Veterans Health Administration. Drug Alcohol Depend. 2017 Jul 11;178:527-533.

be withdrawn from alcohol without much difficulty as outpatients or day-patients. GPs with an interest in the field can easily manage most withdrawals, especially in countries where they have access to hospital beds but alcoholism is no exception to the general rule that in-patient treatment should only be used if out-patient treatment is not appropriate. Disulfiram is particularly effective in helping patients to stay dry in their normal surroundings during the crucial and relapse-prone first few weeks after stopping drinking, despite internal and external temptations. However, for reasons that have more to do with profitability and ideology than with patient choice or the evidence-base, many 'rehabs' and private addiction clinics do not offer either disulfiram or out-patient withdrawal.

When a patient's history or circumstances suggest that he is at high risk of relapse in the first few days or weeks of abstinence and medication seems indicated, that risk will be considerably lower with disulfiram than with other drugs. If clinicians prefer to follow the current official advice in Britain to use those other drugs first but then find that excessive and damaging drinking continues, they should not hesitate before discussing a change to disulfiram. The patient who refused to take disulfiram because 'you're trying to get me to stop drinking' refused precisely because he knew – *without even having taken it himself* - that disulfiram is a very effective drug. You should now know a lot more than he knew and we hope you will have even more respect than he did for a drug that for far too long has been ignored, misrepresented and misunderstood.

Appendix 1. OTHER USES OF DISULFIRAM.

Under the trade-name Tetmosol, monosulfiram is still available in some countries for the treatment of scabies but there are many alternatives, including one – ivermectin – that is often effective with a single oral dose. For bacterial rather than parasitic infections, disulfiram may find a use in the treatment of tuberculosis,[260] where resistant strains make the development of new antibacterial classes a matter of some urgency. It also has antifungal[261] and antiviral[262] properties.

At present, the main non-alcohol interest in disulfiram centres around the anti-cancer effects that are related to its chelating properties.[263] It shows promise as a topical treatment for cervical cancer[264] and when incorporated in biodegradable plastic micro-rods, for glioblastoma multiforme,[265] and cancers of the lung[266] and liver.[267] The

---

[260] Dalecki AG, Haeili M, Shah S, et al. Disulfiram and copper ions kill Mycobacterium tuberculosis in a synergistic manner. Antimicrob Agents Chemother. 2015 Jun 1. pii: AAC.00692-15. [Epub ahead of print]

[261] Khan S, Singhal S, Mathur T. et al. Antifungal potential of disulfiram. Jpn J Med Mycol 2007;48.109-13

[262] Chen SC, Jeng KS,1, Lai MM.Zinc finger-containing cellular transcription corepressor ZBTB25 promotes influenza virus RNA transcription and is a target for zinc-ejector drugs. J Virol. 2017 Aug 2. pii: JVI.00842-17. doi: 10.1128/JVI.00842-17.

[263] Tawari PE, Wang Z, Najlah M, et al The cytotoxic mechanisms of disulfiram and copper(ii) in cancer cells. Toxicol Res (Camb). 2015 Nov 19;4(6):1439-1442.

[264] Baffoe CS, Nguyen N, Boyd P, Wang W, Morris M, McConville C. Disulfiramloaded immediate and extended release vaginal tablets for the localised treatment of cervical cancer. J Pharm Pharmacol. 2014 Dec 10. doi: 10.1111/jphp.12330.

[265] McConville C, Tawari P, Wang W.Hot melt extruded and injection moulded disulfiram-loaded PLGA millirods for the treatment of

same properties may make it useful in the x-linked genetic childhood disorder Menkes' Disease, for which there is currently no effective treatment.[268]

In addition to its use in nickel dermatitis, previously discussed, its chelating qualities make it useful in acute nickel carbonyl poisoning.[269]

Anaesthetists and intensivists may like to know that it seems useful for ketamine cardiotoxicity[270] (at least in rats) while as eye drops, it reduces intra-ocular pressure in rabbits.[271]

---

glioblastoma multiforme via stereotactic injection. Int J Pharm. 2015 Oct 15;494(1):73-82.
[266] Najlah M, Ahmed Z, Iqbal M, Wang Z, Tawari P, Wang W, McConville C. Development and characterisation of disulfiram-loaded PLGA nanoparticles for the treatment of non-small cell lung cancer. Eur J Pharm Biopharm. 2017 Mar;112:224-233. doi: 10.1016/j.ejpb.2016.11.032.
[267] Wang Z, Tan J, McConville C, et al Poly lactic-co-glycolic acid controlled delivery of disulfiram to target liver cancer stem-like cells. Nanomedicine. 2016 Aug 10;13(2):641-657.
[268] Hoshi Y, Tani N, Tabata H, et al. Development of a therapeutic agent for menkes disease: solubilization of a copper-disulfiram complex. Yakugaku Zasshi. 2015;135(3):493-9
[269] Bowman N, Caravati EM, et al. Acute pneumonitis associated with nickel carbonyl exposure in the workplace. Clin Toxicol (Phila). 2017 Jul 28:1-3. doi: 10.1080/15563650.2017.1355057.
[270] Cetin N, Suleyman B, Altuner D, Effect of disulfiram on ketamine-induced cardiotoxicity in rats. Int J Clin Exp Med. 2015 Aug 15;8(8):13540-7. eCollection 2015.
[271] Nagai N, Yoshioka C, Mano Y, Ito Y, et al.Effect of Eye Drops Containing Disulfiram and Low- Substituted Methylcellulose in Reducing Intraocular Pressure in Rabbit Models. Curr Eye Res. 2014 Oct 20:1-11.

Finally, given the excessive anxieties about disulfiram's hepatotoxicity, it is interesting that it protects rats against hepatic necrosis due to paracetamol,[272] (a life-threatening and still not rare complication of paracetamol overdose) though this protection may not extend to humans.[273]

---

[272] Hazai E, Vereczkey L, Monostory K. Reduction of toxic metabolite formation of acetaminophen. Biochem Biophys Res Commun. 2002 Mar 8;291(4):1089-94.
[273] Poulsen HE, Ranek L, Jørgensen L. The influence of disulfiram on acetaminophen metabolism in man. Xenobiotica. 1991 Feb;21(2):243-9.

ACKNOWLEDGEMENTS

The late Doug Anglin of UCLA introduced me to the potential of hair-testing for illicit drugs and, eventually, alcohol. He also gave me a crash course in methadone maintenance when I needed to learn about it very quickly. Peter Bourne, now probably the oldest living major disulfiram researcher since Nathan Azrin died in 2013, provided several interesting and useful insights into the origins of his pioneering 1966 study and into addiction treatment and policy in America more generally. Jonathan Chick of Edinburgh and Duncan Raistrick of the Leeds Addiction Unit, two other persistent British defenders and researchers of disulfiram, read the first draft and we have incorporated most of their suggestions. Morris Faiman of the University of Kansas keeps me posted about the pharmaceutical industry's lack of interest in the functioning implant that he has developed. Yedy Israel of the University of Santiago provided updates about progress with gene-therapy for alcoholism. Henning Krampe of the Charité Hospital, Berlin and Hannelore Ehrenreich of Göttingen's Max Planck Institute discussed the details of their astoundingly successful OLITA programme and allowed me to use some of their illustrations. Haremi Kudo shared his unheralded discovery, as a Japanese adolescent, of the consequences of inheriting inefficient variants of ALDH.

Jan Linssen provided the very latest international research findings about the large and near-universal deterrent effects of speed cameras. Paul McCann and Harry Vann guided me through the process of setting up the book's website. The late John Sawle-Thomas, one of my first and finest teachers, encouraged me, as a very junior psychiatrist, to attend courses on cognitive behavioural and marital therapies because he correctly predicted that they were the psychotherapies of the future and a useful counterforce to the prevalent but already declining Freudian orthodoxies. Without him, I might not have realized how easily, logically and effectively disulfiram can be incorporated into psychosocial treatments.

Neither of us has any conflicts of interest to declare.

INDEX

1

12-step clinics
   and rejection of DSF, 198
12-step groups
   unusual incorporation of DSF by Irish group, 195
12-step movement
   and opposition to medication, 193
12-step treatment
   and opposition to NTX, 196
   unique hegemony of, in USA, 198
12-step treatment and clinics, 40

4

4-methylpyrrazole, 188

A

Abstinence
   as only acceptable goal for AA, 196
   length of previous A- as predictor of future A-, 228
Abstinence violation effect, 139
acamprosate, 79
Acamprosate, xii, 38, 45
Acamprosate (ACP)
   abstinence rate 50% lower than DSF, 221
Accountants, 24, 58
Acetaldehyde
   excretion pathways, 188
Acta Psychiatrica DSF Supplement,, 87
Active placebo, 58
Addiction (journal)
   Editorials in support of DSF, 200
Addiction physicians
   'prominence of recovering addicts' among APs in USA, 198
ADHD, 172
Adlerian psychotherapy, 199
Adverse reactions
   surveillance for, 87
Alcohol
   in-patient withdrawal from, 112
Alcohol challenge
   indications for, 190
   rarity of need for, 185
   technique, 190
Alcohol-detecting tags
   in probation-linked treatment, 131
Alcoholic patients
   varieties of, 33
Alcoholic physicians
   management of, 159
Alcoholics Anonymous, 76
   adverse comparisons with other self-help groups, 193
Alcoholics Anonymous (AA), 35
Alcoholism
   as generic term, xvii
   high mortality of, 77
   mortality of in Britain, 240
   social causes of changes in incidence, 209
Alcohol-related injuries, 43
Aldehyde dehydrogenase (ALDH)
   as cause of DAR, 4
   sub-types, 27
ALDH
   in East Asians, 28
   in non-Japanese populations, 28
   representation of differing genotypes, 28
   variable length of inhibition by DSF, 150

ALDH inhibition
  persistence of, 15
ALDH2*1, 27
ALDH2*2/*2, 29
Alho H, 63, 73
Ambivalence, 9
  about DSF among non-medical health professionals, 197
Amish, 27
Antabuse, xi, 5
Anticonvulsants
  no need for routine prescribing of in withdrawal, 113
Anti-craving effects
  of ACP and NTX not reflected in better outcomes, 221
Anti-craving medicines, 64
Antidepressants
  excessive and inappropriate prescribing of, 115
  limited effectiveness of, 58
Antihistamines, 189
Anxiety management, 138
Archbishop of Canterbury, 118
Aspirin
  DSF 'safer than', 171
Assertive aftercare
  important feature of OLITA, 142
Assertiveness training, 38
Atlanta DSF programme
  and few AEs despite poor health of patients, 121
  and good results in unpromising patients, 121
Attribution theory, 76
Automaticity
  of alcohol-free responses as aim of DSF treatment, 144
Autonomy
  restored by DSF, 239
Azrin N et al, 21

B

Baseline testing
  for court reports, 162
Benzodiazepine loading technique
  in alcohol withdrawal, 113
Berglund M, 63, 65
Bickel et al, 31
Bioavailability
  differing bioavailability of different DSF tablets, 81
  variable, of DSF, 111
Biomedical explanations, 53
Blood tests, 56
  questionable need for, before starting DSF, 88
Blood-brain barrier, 182
Bourne, Peter
  and background to Atlanta probation-linked DSF study, 119
  and first probation-linked DSF study, 119
Brain damage
  in alcoholism, testing for, 163
Brain disease hypothesis in addictions
  implications of DSF for, 207
Brain disease model
  and failure to explain recovery, 210
Breathalyser
  usefulness of, in starting DSF, 108
Buprenorphine
  in combination with DSF, 103

C

Carbohydrate-Deficient Transferrin, 160
Care proceedings, 161
Celebrity rehabs, 33, 240
Chan KY.
  and Singapore NTX probation study, 67
Changi Prison
  and effective NTX programme, 130

Charisma, 59
Chelating
  properties of DSF, 2
Chelation
  of DSF with nickel, 173
Chick J, 63, 64
  and contribution of ritual to DSF effectivness, 204
Children of alcoholics
  may or may not develop alcoholism, 209
Chlordiazepoxide, 124
Cirrhosis of the liver
  life-saving role of DSF in, 180
Clinical psychologists
  prominent in DSF research, 24
Cognitive behavioural therapy, 69
Colorado Springs
  and 13-fold reduction in offending with DSF, 124
COMBINE study
  minimal effects of ACP and NTX vs placebo, 216
Community reinforcement model, 10
Community Reinforcement Therapy, 25
Complementary and Alternative medicine, 53
Compliance, 9, 218, 227
Components of treatment, 49
Compulsory treatment
  difficulties of, in alcoholism, 90
Contra-indications to DSF
  few and mostly relative, 115
Controlled drinking, 42, 54
  after DSF treatment, 204
Copenhagen
  round table symposium on DSF, 63
  wartime scabies epidemic in, 1
Copenhagen Round Table Symposium, xv
Copenhagen symposium, 171
Coping skills
  importance of practising in real life, 139
Cost-effectiveness, 38, 241
counselling
  large variations in effectiveness of, 59
Counselling
  not always necessary, 37
Couples therapy, 14
Court of Appeal, 163
Crisis interventions
  in OLITA, 141
Cue exposure, 137
Cue-exposure, 138
Cyanamide, 101, 175
  as alternative to DSF, 3
  for 'temperance therapy' in Japan, 151
  in Canada, 76
  in skin patch test for ALDH inhibition, 191

D

da Silva A.
  and comparative studies against ACP and NTX, 221
DAR, 49
  in early use of DSF, 5
  vicarious knowedge of, 49
Delirium tremens
  dangers of herbal remedies and 'culturally sensitive' treatment., 122
  importance of benzodiazepines in preventing, 112
  inappropriateness of anti-psychotic drugs in, 113
Depot naltrexone
  and marginal advantage over placebo injection, 219
Depot-naltrexone
  and failure to reduce methamphetamine abuse, 221

lack of very heavy drinkers in
many RCTs, 218
Depression
in dual diagnosis, 57
vs understandable misery, 117
Deterrence
effectiveness of in reducing
truancy, 205
ideological opposition to, 205
Deterrent effect of DAR, 31
Deterrent effect of DSF
equally effective with or without
family history, 212
Detoxification, 68
Diazepam, 113
Difficult patients, 33
Directly Observed Treatment', 10
Disease model of alcoholism, 53
disulfiram
and drug interactions, 184
and probation-linked treatment,
119
Disulfiram
17 years treatment record, 41
adverse effects (AEs) of, 171
adverse interaction with
metronidazole, 184
and 'average' level of adverse
effects, 92
and 'difficult' patients, 240
and 2x/wk or 3x/wk dosing, 114
and active metabolite, 81
and bioilar disorder, 118
and bipolar disorder, 94
and buprenorphine, 103
and cardiovascular disease, 183
and chelation, 181
and confusional states
possible mechanisms, 182
and dose increases, 82
and drug interactions, 82
and general compatibility with
psychotropic medication,
184
and group therapy, 83
and how quickly to start, 108

and lithium, 118
and nickel, 95
and nickel dermatitis, 91
and pregnancy, 184
and skin reactions, 90
and stimulants for persistent
tiredness as AE, 172
and superiority to CBT or 12-
step facilitation, 223
and teratogenicity, 89
and the foetus, 88
and the liver, 87
anti-cancer effects, 243
as aid to controlled drinking,
150
as pro-drug, 4, 111
as vermicide, 2
contraindications, 98
current NHS advice on, 242
differing bioavailability of, 97
dosage of, 80
duration of treatment, 41
early recognition that DSF
'paves the way for
psychotherapy', 6
educational mechanism of
effects, 210
empowering effects of, 52
exaggerated dangers of, 240
first synthesized in 1881, 1
for detoxified opiate users who
drink heavily despite taking
NTX, 167
hepatotoxicity, 245
importance of adequate dosage,
159
in alcoholic methadone
maintenance patients, 164
in Austria, 66
in cocaine abuse, 95, 166
in Denmark, 80, 90, 180
in Finland, 73
in high risk situations, 149
in Italy, 68
in methadone maintenance, 101,
124

in Norway, 74
in pregnancy, 88
in rubber industry, 1
in schizophrenia, 94, 96
in Sweden, 65
in tuberculosis treatment, 243
is not 'aversion therapy', 203
metabolism in liver disease, 83
mis-labelled as aversion
 therapy, 5
mortality of treatment, 92
need for dose increases, 40, 51
overdoses of, 95
possible lack of DAR in serious
 liver disease, 81
prevents endless internal
 arguments, 239
probation-linked, 60
prolonged action of, 17
psychotic reactions to, 97
rarity of psychotic reactions to,
 98
reduces ruminations, 239
revival of, 24
safety in psychotic patients, 94
selection of patients for, 107
sexual side-effects of, 69
short-term treatment with, 68
starting dose, 110
superiority to ACP and NTX in
 Finnish study, 222
surreptitious use of, 72
targeted or intermittent use, 204
the correct dose is 'enough', 192
underprescribing of, 241
unique problems in RCTs, 20
unsupervised studies, 23
use with acamprosate or
 naltrexone, 99
vs other medications for
 alcoholism, 215
Disulfiram challenge
 to confirm cause of hepatitis,
 177
Disulfiram hepatitis
 avoidability of, 176

early signs and symptoms of,
 177
incidence of, 176
timing and features of, 176
unexpectedly high proportion of
 female patients, 91
Disulfiram hepatotoxicity, 91
Disulfiram implants
 and ethical dilemmas, 232
 and increased effects of injected
  placebos, 227
 and lack of ALDH inhibition,
  227
 and undetectable blood levels of
  DSF, 82
 and unsuitability of depot
  injections, 231
 ineffective but can cause
  fulminating DSF hepatitis,
  229
 reasons for lack of
  pharmacological effect, 229
Disulfiram neuropathy
 relationship to DSF dose, 174
 reversibility of, 93
 timing and features of, 175
Disulfiram-alcohol reaction
 observing in clinic, 85
Disulfiram-Alcohol Reaction
 colour photographs of, on
  website, 186
 factors influencing severity of,
  186
 importance of emphasising
  risks, 187
 rarity of deaths from, 187
 varying attitudes of patients to,
  186
Disulfiram-Alcohol Reaction
 (DAR)., 1
Dopamine β-hydroxylase
 inhibition by DSF, 183
Dopamine-beta-hydroxylase,, 31
Dosage
 of DSF, 31
Drip, 138

Drug-placebo differences
    for anti-depressants, mainly small, 117
Dual diagnosis', 116
    improvements in with DSF, 141
Dumex, 63

E

Early-warning system
    unique to DSF, 15
Easy patients, 33
ECG
    not usually urgent need for, 115
Edwards *et al*
    treatment vs advice study, 21
Edwards G
    and spontaneous improvement, 33
Edwards G.
    and hostility to DSF, 200
EEG abnormalities
    in DSF confusional state, 182
Effect size
    double for DSF vs ACP and NTX, 220
Ehrenreich, Dr Hannelore. *See* OLITA
Empowerment
    increased by DSF, 239
Enghusen-Poulsen H, 63
Enzyme inhibition
    in white blood cells, 84
Ethics, 38
    of DSF treatment, 193
Ethyl glucuronide, 161
Evasion
    techniques used by patients, 12
Evidence-based interventions
    treatment menu of, 107
Experts
    'automatic problem-solving is cjaracteristic mode of, 144
Exposure and response-prevention
    as major mechanism of DSF effectiveness, 139

Exposure and Response-Prevention (ERP), 137

F

Faiman, Prof M
    and effective implants, 230
Families
    involvement in treatment, 75
Family courts, 161
Family therapy, 79
Fear and loathing in Westminster.
    See website: planetservetus.com
Foetal alcohol syndrome, 184
Foreign, 139
Foreign language-learning analogy, 56
Fox, Ruth, 154
Fraser McLuskey, Rev.
    the parachute padre, as supervisor, 127
Freud S.
    and self-medication with cocaine, 200
Fuller *et al*, 41, 80
Fuller *et al* 1986
    misleading RCT, 20
Functional polymorphism
    of mu-opioid receptor gene, 217

G

Galanter, 42
Galanter M
    and family therapy, 76
    and network therapy, 41
Gamma glutyl transpetidase, 160
Gamma-hydroxybutyrate, 102
Geerlings P, 63, 73, 80
Gene therapy for alcoholism, 235
General practitioners, 70, 74
Geneva group
    and alleged general irrationality of all addicts, 204
    and alleged lack of theoretical justification for DSF, 200

and ethical objections to DSF, 201
refutation of arguments of, 203
George Best and DSF implants, 232
Getz, Stan
  DSF featuring in divorce proceedings of, 152
Golfers
  expert vs less expert, significant differences in brain activity of, 144
Gossop M
  criticises brain disease model, 207
GPs
  managing alcohol withdrawal, 242

H

Habits
  difficulty of changing in alcoholism, 136
Hair testing
  for alcohol metabolites, 163
  for alcoholic physicians, 161
Hald J., 3
Hardt F, 63
Haynes
  and probation-linked DSF study, 129
Healthy complier effect', 55
Hepatitis C
  DSF's usefulness in treating, 181
heterozygotes, 28
High-risk situations, 70
Homozygosity
  alcoholism extremely rare in, 30
Homozygous, 27
Hostels, 17
Hydrogen sulphide
  as metabolite of DSF, 173
Hypnotics
  attitudes to prescribing in alcohol withdrawal, 112
Hypotension
  in DAR, 85

I

Immersion methods
  of foreign language-learning, 136

J

Jacobsen E., 2
Jaundice
  need to warn patients about significance of, 92
Johnsen J, 63
Jung C., 199

K

Kalant H
  and criticism of brain disease model, 210
Kleinian psychotherapy, 199
Koreans, 28
Krampe, Dr Henning. *See* OLITA

L

Lapse
  vs relapse, 15
Lapses
  vs 'relapses', 145
  vs relapses, 46
Larson at al
  safety of DSF in psychiatric disorders, 94
Lead poisoning, sub-clinical
  possible mechanism of confusional states with DSF in India, 182
Learning
  as, 211
Lesch O, 63, 66, 69

and typology of alcoholism, 79
Leshner A
 and brain disease model, 208
Lewis M.
 and critique of brain disease model, 210
Liebson and Faillace
 linking DSF to prescribed benzodiazepines, 123
Listerine
 alarmist attitudes to, 238
Lithium
 and DSF, 118
Liver function tests
 non-pathological abnormalities in, 180
Liver function tests (LFTs)., 35
Liver funtion tests
 in fulminating hepatitis, 229
Liver toxicity. See Ch 14 Side effects
Locus of control
 external vs internal, doubtful relevance of, 188
Lorazepam, 113

M

Maladaptive
 behaviour and responses, 137
Malignant relapse, 142
MAOI-inhibitors
 compatibility of DSF with, 185
Marathons
 as cause of raised LFTs, 180
Marital Therapy, 16
Markers of alcohol abuse, 160
Martensen-Larsen, O, 3
Martenson-Larsen, O, 64
Mean Corpuscular Volume (MCV), 160
Meta-analyses
 consistently show DSF superior to NTX and ACP, 215
Metronidazole
 adverse reaction with DSF, 184
Miller W.
and narrow views of 12-step counsellors, 197
Miller WR.
 support for DSF, 24
Mini-lapse, 142
Minnesota-model treatment, 77
Monitoring techniques
 for treatment compliance, 160
Monoclonal antibodies
 as treatment for chemical addictions, 231
Monosulfiram
 in scabies treatment, 243
Morphine
 with DSF, as alternative to methadone, 165
Motivational interviewing, 10

N

Nalmefene, xii, 180
Naltrexone, 45
 and damage limitation in alcoholim, 79
 and failure to prevent heavy drinking, 224
 and ineffectiveness in combined alcohol and cocaine abuse, 223
 clinically insignificant differences compared with placebo, 217
 greater effectiveness in opiate abuse than in alcoholism, 196
 heroin-blocking role, xvi
 probation-linked treatment with, in Westminster, 130
 safety of in liver disease, 168
 usefulness of long-acting preparations in opiate abuse, 227
Naltrexone implants
 and therapeutic strategies, 231
Network therapy, 84
Neuroadaptive changes
 universality of, 208

Neuroimaging studies
   and cerebral plasticity, 212
Neuronal circuits
   in addiction, 207
Neuropathological changes
   due to alcohol, 212
New Zealand study, 50, 53
   and DSF dose increases, 146
New Zealand study), 56
Newton-Howes et al, 31, 50
NHS, 74
Nichts über die zunge', 193
Nickel, 173
Nickel allergy
   and DSF, 96
Nickel-sensitivity
   causes of, 179
   importance of asking about, 179
   in Denmark, incidence of, 179
Non-specific and placebo effects
   in psychotherapies, 213
Null hypothesis, xiii

O

Obsessive-compulsive patients
   and response-prevention, 137
OLITA, 42, 46, 140
   and unique 9-year follow-up, 143
   and optimum length of DSF treatment, 143
   unpromising characteristics of patient group, 140
OLITA programme, 17
Oriental flush, 28, 189

P

Patient education
   about side effects, importance of, 177
Patient information leaflets, 75
Patients
   unpredictability of, when first entering treatment, 39

Patient-therapist relationship, 59
Perceptions
   of clinicians, 57
   of patients, 57
Peripheral neuropathy, 87
Personality traits, 55
Pharmaceutical industry
   and lack of funding for DSF research, 198
Pharmacokinetics
   of DSF, 84
Phillips M
   and subcutaneous DSF sludge, 230
Philosophy
of DSF treatment, 193
physical examinations, 56
Placebo, xiv, 22, 51, 55, 57
   active, 58
   deliberate prescribing of, 60
Placebo and non-specific effects, 53, 57
   importance in alcoholism treatment generally, 35
   in DSF treatment, 49
Placebo DSF, 32
Placebo injections, 218
   only 25% less effective than depot NTX, 218
Poldrugo F, 63
Politics
of DSF treatment, 193
positive reinforcement'
   vs deterrence, 205
Priests, 10, 17, 56
private practice, 38
Probation officers, 10
Probation-linked disulfiram, 162
Problem-oriented interventions, 17
Prochaska and DiClemente model, 50
Pseudo-bars, 138
Psychiatrists
   and failure to notice AEs of DSF, 177
Psychoanalysis

residual influence of, 199

R

Randomised Controlled Trial, 57
RCT, xiv
Randomised controlled trial (RCT)., 20
Recurrent alcohol-related offenders, 60
Recurrent alcohol-related offenders
   predicted superiority of DSF vs depot NTX, 219
Refusal
   of treatment, 38
Regression to the mean, 56, 116
Relapse, 37
   as emergency, 141
Relapse prevention, 39
Religious aspects of treatment, 56
Residential rehabs
   and irrational relapse policies, 196
   artificial atmosphere of, 139
   high cost of, 109
Response-prevention, 137
Reward pathways, 209
ruminations, 52
Ruminations, 52

S

Saliva alcohol test-strips, 108
Salvation Army hostels, 127
Sauces
   alcohol in, 30
Saunders B, 24
Scabies
   effectiveness of DSF in, 2
Self-help groups, 54
Serendipity
   in discovery of DSF's actions, 1
Sereny et al, 39
   DSF study, 134
Serious alcohol-related offences
   pre-trial investigations and management, 162
   usefulness of brain scans in investigations for, 162
Shaw, George Bernard
   on faith in doctors, 75
Sinclair Method of alcoholism treatment
   superiority of targeted DSF to, 222
Singapore
   and probation-linked NTX in heroin-related offenders, 130
Skid-row alcoholics
   predominant patient group in Atlanta study, 120
Skin test
   for ALDH inhibition, 191
Skinner et al meta-analysis, 220
Skinner M.
   important meta-analysis, 22
Slow release oral morphine
   and DSF, 165
S-methyl N,N-diethylthiolcarbamate sulfoxide, 230
   active metabolite of DSF, 4
Social re-integration
   in OLITA, 141
Social structure, 53
Social workers, 77
Speed cameras, xiv, 203
Spider-phobia, 137
SSRIs
   lack of effect on drinking, 100
Starting dose
   of DSF, 110
State-funded treatment, 38
Style
   of counsellors and therapists, importance of, 16
Submersion methods
   of foreign language-learning, 137
Supervised disulfiram
   as crucial component of OLITA, 141

Supervision, 11
Swallowing
 of DSF, importance of observing, 13
Sydenham, xii
Symptom substitution
 as alleged consequence of CBT, 199

T

Tablet substitution
 as evasion technique, 14
Temperance therapy', 151
Temptation, 52
Teratogenicity
 and DSF, 184
The 'Five Ds'
 Divorce, Dismissal, Debt, De-housing, Death, 107
The Netherlands
 predominance of heroin smoking vs injecting in, 209
Theoretical orientation
 of counsellors and psychotherapists, 59
Therapist rotation
 important feature of OLITA, 142
Thorens G.. See Geneva group
Thought-suppression
 counter-productivity of, 214
Treatment vs Advice
 important British study, 34
Truancy
 effectiveness of deterrence in, 205

U

Unconscious problems
 allegedly underlying alcoholism, 199
Underlying problems

 often a result of alcoholism, not a cause, 199
University of Chile bibulous rats', 235
Unmotivated patients, 43

V

Vertebroplasty, 58, 59
Vietnam
 and US heroin addicts, 209
Vitamin C, 189
Volkow N.
 and brain disease model of addictions, 207
Vomiting
 as evasion technique, 13

W

Westminster Hospital, 125
Westminster probation-linked DSF programme
 attitude of magistrates to, 128
 origins of, 128
 results of, published in BMJ, 129
Wilson, Bill
 inclusive and tolerant attitude of AA founder, 194
Withdrawal from alcohol
 appropriate regimes for, 112
 as in-patient, rarely needs >4-5 days, 114
World Health Organization
 recommends inclusion of DSF, 105

Z

Zierau J, 63, 68
Zullino D. See Geneva group

www.ingramcontent.com/pod-product-compliance
Lightning Source LLC
Chambersburg PA
CBHW050200230526
45470CB00001B/170